Alcohol Problems in the Community

Edited by Larry Harrison

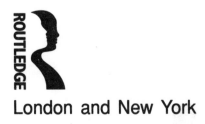
ROUTLEDGE

London and New York

First published 1996
by Routledge
11 New Fetter Lane, London EC4P 4EE

Simultaneously published in the USA and Canada
by Routledge
29 West 35th Street, New York, NY 10001

Typeset in Times by Florencetype Ltd, Stoodleigh, Devon
Printed and Bound in Great Britain by Mackays of
Chatham PLC, Chatham, Kent

British Library Cataloguing in Publication Data
A catalogue record for this book is available from the
British Library

Library of Congress Cataloguing in Publication Data
A catalogue record for this book has been requested

ISBN 0-415-11042-4 (hbk)
ISBN 0-415-11043-2 (pbk)

Contents

Illustrations

Contributors

Victor Adebowale is one of only two Black directors of mainstream housing organisations. He has been Director of the Alcohol Recovery Project, London, since 1990, and established *Choices*, the Black Alcohol Centre, in 1993.

Roy Carr-Hill is a Senior Research Fellow at the Centre for Health Economics at the University of York.

William R. Downs is Professor of Social Work and Director of the Center for the Study of Adolescence at the University of Northern Iowa.

Emma Fossey has been a member of the Alcohol Research Group at the University of Edinburgh since 1990.

Anna Green is a researcher at the Centre for the Study of Drugs and Health Behaviour, London.

Philip Guy is Student Unit Manager at the Hull and East Yorkshire Council for Drug Problems.

Larry Harrison has been a researcher at the University of Hull's Institute for Health Studies since 1983. He was a member of the Economic and Social Research Council's Addiction Research Centre 1983–85, and appointed Senior Lecturer in Social Work at the University of Hull in 1992.

Mary Harrison is a Lecturer in Social Work at the University of York and Coordinator of the Black External Assessors Association.

Wendy Loretto is a social scientist and has been a member of the Alcohol Research Group at the University of Edinburgh since

1991. She was appointed Lecturer in the Department of Business Studies at the University of Edinburgh in 1994.

Hugo Luck qualified as a social worker at the University of Hull where he is currently working as a doctoral student, studying the evaluation of community and hospital-based services for people with drinking problems.

Jill Manthorpe is a Lecturer in Community Care at the University of Hull.

Roger Marshall as a Social Worker at the Alcohol and Substance Misuse Team, London Road, Sheffield.

Brenda A. Miller is Deputy Director of the New York State Institute for the Study of Addictions, Buffalo, NY.

Martin Plant is Director of the Alcohol Research Group and Professorial Fellow at the University of Edinburgh.

Wayne Sivyer is Senior Social Work Practitioner at the Drugs, Alcohol Resource Team, Hull.

Betsy Thom is a Head of Training at the Centre for the Study of Drugs and Health Behaviour, London.

Jan Waterson is a Lecturer in Social Services Management at the Department of Social Policy and Social Work, the University of Birmingham.

Acknowledgements

I am grateful to Dorothy Vahid-Kasiri for preparing this text for publication, and to the Journal of Studies on Alcohol for agreeing to the reproduction of Tables 1.7 and 1.8 in Chapter 1. These were originally published in an article by Brenda A. Miller, William R. Downs and Maria Testa entitled 'Interrelationships between victimisation experiences and women's alcohol/drug use', in the *Journal of Studies on Alcohol* 1993, supplement 12, 109–17.

I am also grateful to Helen Gould, information officer at the former Yorkshire Regional Health Authority, for providing the hospital activity statistics which are analysed in Chapter 3. Special thanks are due to Mathew Sutton, research fellow at the Centre for Health Economics, University of York, who is collaborating with me on an analysis of alcohol-related mortality statistics by country of birth, and who did much of the preliminary work on this data set. Thanks also to Steve Southall for his comments on homelessness.

Emma Fossey, Wendy Loretto and Martin Plant are indebted to colleagues and former members of the Alcohol Research Group for assistance in the production of their review. In particular Drs Carl May and Deborah Lister Sharp are acknowledged. Their review was supported by the Portman Group, the Scotch Whisky Association and the Alcohol Education and Research Council.

William R. Downs and Brenda A. Miller wish to express their appreciation to the agencies who allowed access to their clients, and especially to the women who shared their stories with them. Their research was funded in part by the US National Institute on Alcohol Abuse and Alcoholism, NIH, Grant No. R01AA07554.

Introduction

Community surveys reveal large numbers of people drinking at high risk levels, typically about 6 per cent of the adult male and 1 per cent of the adult female population in England and Wales (see, e.g., Goddard and Ikin 1988). At a conservative estimate, this means that something like 800,000 people are at risk of developing alcohol-related problems, at least one-third of whom are already exhibiting symptoms of alcohol dependence. A disproportionate number of these problem drinkers show up in primary health care, social work and probation practice, although they are rarely identified as such (Shaw *et al.* 1978; Jarman and Kellett 1979; Abel 1983).

Alarming though the extent of unrecognised alcohol-related morbidity may seem, it does not necessarily indicate the need for a massive expansion of specialist services. Nor does it mean that primary care staff should take on a specialist task. The large numbers of problem drinkers identified in community surveys have different characteristics from the minority who seek treatment (Room 1977). Those seen by alcohol treatment agencies are usually men aged 40–55 years, with poor employment records, marked relationship difficulties and co-existing physical and mental health problems. Those identified in community surveys are also typically male, but are likely to be much younger, to have a history of social stability, and are less likely to be experiencing health-related problems.

There are similar findings for depression and anxiety-related disorders (Goldberg and Huxley 1992). Most people who experience an episode of depression or neurosis do not consult a medical practitioner over their symptoms; many of those who do seek help are not recognised as having a mental disorder; and only a minority of those who are recognised as having a disorder are referred to specialist psychiatric services. Perhaps not surprisingly, such people are more likely to be suffering from severe disorders, like schizophrenia, or to have more entrenched problems (Goldberg and Huxley 1992).

Similarly, those who reach the specialist alcohol treatment agencies are more likely to have severe problems, and represent the extreme end of a continuum. It has been known for some time from general population surveys that the distribution of alcohol consumption is continuous and uni-modal: there is no evidence for the existence of two populations of consumers, the normal and the abnormal. The epidemiological evidence also suggests that there is a wide range of problems associated with alcohol consumption – with the number and kinds of disabilities increasing progressively with the amount of alcohol consumed (Bruun *et al.* 1975; Edwards *et al.* 1994).

While it is possible to identify at-risk behaviour, it is difficult to assign individuals into fixed categories of social drinker, heavy drinker and 'true alcoholic'. Retrospective and longitudinal studies indicate that most problem drinkers move into and out of periods of dependent drinking, although the duration and severity of these episodes vary (Cahalan and Room 1974; Vaillant and Milofsky 1982). Rather than there being a clearly defined category of 'alcoholic', many of those judged to be alcohol dependent will return to controlled or asymptomatic drinking (Heather 1987; Heather and Robertson 1983; Miller 1983; Sanchez-Craig *et al.* 1984).

This is in marked contrast to the earlier view of alcohol dependence as a progressive and irreversible disease – a view which still has many adherents. Controversy over the nature of drinking problems will doubtless continue, with some arguing to retain a modified disease concept, while others debate whether there could be two types of alcohol dependence – an intractable and genetically transmitted variety and a less severe, environmentally determined kind (Cloninger *et al.*, 1981; Vaillant 1994). The view which is gaining ground in the UK, however, whether derived from a bio-psycho-social or a cognitive-behavioural model (Rollnick 1985; Levin 1990), stresses the continuity of normal and abnormal behaviour.

This reflects the shift in social psychiatry from a categorical to a *dimensional* view of common mental disorders; that is, from a concern with taxonomy, with the classification and sub-classification of symptoms into discrete disease entities, to a perception that common mental health problems are multi-dimensional (Goldberg and Huxley 1992). From this perspective, there are no rigid boundaries between normal and pathological populations, nor between common diagnostic categories. Rather than determine whether or not individuals fall within particular diagnostic categories, it may be more important to establish the extent to which they have psychological problems.

This growing appreciation of the essential unity of mundane, everyday, commonplace psychological problems and the more extreme manifestations of mental distress has focused attention on resilience. In most cases, common mental disorders are resolved within a matter of weeks, without professional help. It is usually when the normal process of remission is impaired or delayed for some reason that people are referred to psychiatric services (Goldberg and Huxley 1992).

Most of those identified in community surveys as having alcohol-related disabilities will also resolve their problems without intervention. Professional help can often hasten the remission process, however, and evidence is accumulating for the success of brief, low-cost interventions, particularly with non-treatment-seeking populations (Heather 1987; Hodgson 1989; Miller 1992; Bien et al., 1993; Heather 1994). This is particularly significant for primary health and social care staff, who can be trained in brief interventions as part of their professional qualifying training (see, for example, Harrison 1993b).

In order for brief interventions to be effective it is important to understand not just the factors which destabilise and provoke crisis but those which foster remission or – to use a less clinical term – restitution, the process of losing symptoms (Goldberg and Huxley 1992). Increasingly, in the UK and Australia, the emphasis is on removing impediments to the process of restitution. There is a shift away from deterministic models to those which stress the individual's readiness to change.

The widespread adoption of Prochaska and DiClemente's (1986) model, in particular, has enabled primary care staff to make strategic choices over intervention: from harm minim-isation for those not contemplating change, to techniques aimed at supporting decision-making for those contemplating action, to relapse prevention training for those who have managed to modify their behaviour (Davidson *et al.*, 1991). Rather than reject many problem drinkers as 'unmotivated', there is increasing use of cognitive-behavioural approaches aimed at resolving ambivalence and enhancing motivation (Miller and Rollnick 1991).

It is impossible to over-estimate the importance of this shift in thinking for primary care staff. Until the 1980s, it was usual for alcohol treatment agencies to have rigorous selection procedures, designed to screen out those who lacked motivation, or were otherwise held to have a poor prognosis (Royal College of Psychiatrists 1979: 130). Social workers and others who worked with the most marginalised groups in society – those who rarely met these selection criteria – were working with people who seemed to be hopeless cases, and it was hard for this role to be seen in a positive light (Spratley *et al.*, 1977).

There is now much more optimism about the therapeutic role of social workers, probation officers, and community-based physicians and nurses. Current thinking accepts that most problem drinkers and drug users are likely to feel ambivalent about changing their behaviour. It favours the use of active interventions to engage clients in treatment, and enables front-line professionals to match interventions to the stage of change. This has done much to counter the therapeutic pessimism which inhibited primary level staff in previous years (Shaw *et al.*, 1978). Even when dealing with complex cases which need specialist intervention, primary level staff can employ techniques like brief motivational interviewing to enhance the likelihood of successful referral (Rollnick *et al.*, 1992).

There have also been advances in the prevention of alcohol and drug-related harm, although here progress has been slowest. At a national level, it is possible to identify three modest but fragile successes. These are the reduction in smoking prevalence among adults; the decline in the practice of drinking and driving; and the success of harm-reduction measures aimed at preventing the spread of HIV/AIDS among injecting drug users. No-one would wish to be complacent about any of these achievements – the persistence of cigarette smoking among teenagers and the poorest socioeconomic groups is clearly a source of concern – yet anyone who predicted in 1964 that the prevalence of smoking among adult males would decline by over 20 per cent in the next thirty years would have been dismissed as a fool.

The case of smoking is instructive because cigarette prices, one of the main determinants of consumption, went down in real terms for much of this period (Godfrey and Harrison 1990). Cigarette consumption should have increased as prices fell: instead it declined steadily, probably in response to changing public perceptions of the health risks. Surveys show that in 1964 only 43 per cent of the public accepted that smoking was linked to lung cancer; by the late 1980s this had increased to 80 per cent (Gallup 1976; National Opinion Polls 1984). Government health-promotion activity was minimal for most of this time, and much of the shift in risk perception was probably due to the anti-smoking publicity generated by professional bodies, like the Royal College of Physicians, and to the advice offered individual patients by general medical practitioners and other primary health care staff (Harrison 1989).

The fact that it is possible for front-line professionals to succeed in influencing the smoking habit (tobacco is, after all, widely regarded as the most addictive substance on earth) suggests that there is considerable potential to modify high-risk drinking behaviours at a local level. Despite the existence of detailed studies exploring local opportunities for prevention (Tether and Robinson 1986), and demonstrating how creative prevention programmes have been introduced in some localities (Robinson et al., 1989), local initiatives have yet to make a significant impact on national rates of alcohol-related problems – with the single exception of drinking and driving.

This is significant, because even the most cursory examination of UK government policy shows that the only aspect of alcohol education to have received substantial funding, and where an unambiguous, readily intelligible message has been promoted, is in relation to drinking and driving (Harrison 1989). Local action on drinking and driving, including high-profile law enforcement campaigns in some English counties, has been backed by massive national publicity. Local action to enforce liquor licensing laws, or to enforce local bylaws on street drinking, have also led on occasion to a substantial fall in levels of public disorder and offences by young people – as Emma Fossey, Wendy Loretto and Martin Plant note in Chapter 2 of this book. It is clear that we have only just begun to tap the potential of local prevention activity, and to understand how this should best be supported at a national level.

These recent advances in treatment and prevention are enabling primary health and social care staff to take a lead in responding to drinking problems, something which has been government policy for many years (DHSS and the Welsh Office 1978; DHSS 1981). For these advances in knowledge and skills to become integrated into mainstream professional practice they need to be disseminated through changes to professional education and training, which has always neglected such subjects in the past (Glass 1989; Harrison 1992a). It is notoriously difficult to influence the qualifying training of doctors, nurses and social workers, but medical educators in the US have demonstrated that it can be done, given well-funded curriculum development projects, government incentives to schools of medicine, nursing and social work, and support from validating bodies (Alaszewski and Harrison 1992; Lewis 1989).

In the UK, progress in influencing the professional curriculum has been limited. There have been changes, however, to the qualifying training of social workers and and probation officers, designed to improve their alcohol-related knowledge and skills (Harrison 1992b, 1993a; Scottish Office 1993). Several social work qualifying courses are now providing students with extensive training on substance problems – in one case amounting to over eight weeks of full-time instruction (Harrison 1993b).

The role of social workers and probation officers has also been enhanced by a growing realisation of the importance of social factors in conferring vulnerability to alcohol-related problems. Social class, gender and race are major factors effecting the distribution of tobacco, alcohol and drug-related problems (Cahalan and Room 1974; Pearson 1987; Graham 1993; Harrison et al., 1993; Marsh and McKay 1994), just as they are related to marked inequalities in the prevalence of mortality, and of most physical and psychiatric morbidity (Brown and Harris 1978; Cochrane and Stopes-Roe 1980; Townsend and Davidson 1982). Social structural factors like poor housing, low income, or unemployment, expose some groups to persistent and extreme stress, while limiting access to the material, psychological and social resources required for coping with adversity (Cochrane 1983).

Potentially, at least, interventions aimed at improving social circumstances could make a major impact on alcohol-related problems. But there has been relatively little research on social interventions, despite Vaillant's (1983) finding that US probation

officers who provided alcohol-dependent parolees with supervision, support for job-seeking, and accommodation had more
success than in-patient treatment programmes. There is, however,
a growing research literature on the risks that alcohol poses for
the vulnerable individuals who constitute such a large proportion
of the caseloads of social workers, general medical practitioners
and community based nurses. There have also been a number of
recent innovations in service delivery which deserve to be more
widely known.

This book was written to address the relationship between
social factors such as poverty, homelessness, racism and gender-
based discrimination, and the prevalence and incidence of drinking problems. It does not just seek to document these issues,
however, but to explore the implications for mainstream community services. In cases where services are less developed,
the chapters are the result of collaboration by both social
scientists and practitioners. Where services are more developed,
contributors report the latest research findings. This book will
be of great interest to social work and probation practitioners
and students, therefore, but given the scarcity of literature
examining the social dimensions of drinking problems it should
also be of interest to general medical practitioners, nurses,
police officers and others with an interest in alcohol-related
problems.

The first chapter focuses on child abuse. One of the most
complex and fraught tasks facing community agencies is child
protection. It is surprising – given the level of concern around
child abuse and neglect – that there has been virtually no research
in Europe on the relationship between alcohol and childhood
physical and sexual abuse. In Chapter 1, William Downs and
Brenda Miller report on recent US research on the role of alcohol
in the perpetration of child abuse, and on drinking problems as
a long-term consequence of childhood maltreatment. They show
that an understanding of alcohol problems is actually central to
one of the core social work tasks: child protection. Not only is
there a complex relationship between drinking problems and the
perpetration of abuse, but many of those who have been abused
in childhood develop drinking problems in late adolescence or,
more usually, in adulthood.

There have been periodic 'moral panics' about adolescent
drinking in recent years, even at times when the volume of alcohol

being consumed by young people was stable or declining. Emma Fossey, Wendy Loretto and Martin Plant review recent research on young people's drinking in Chapter 2. They trace changing perceptions of alcohol from childhood to adolescence, and document the different drinking habits of those under 21 in England, Wales, Scotland and Northern Ireland. The authors place the response to the drinking problems experienced by a minority of youths within the normative context of the heavy drinking which has always taken place amongst younger people. They conclude by suggesting which preventive and control measures are likely to be effective with adolescent problem drinkers.

People are, of course, vulnerable to drinking problems at both ends of the life span. In Chapter 3, Larry Harrison, Jill Manthorpe and Roy Carr-Hill demonstrate that the prevalence of drinking problems amongst older people has been under-estimated, and the future implications for community care ignored. Alcohol-related disorders which go unrecognised in the community are more likely to be diagnosed amongst older patients when they are admitted to hospital for other conditions, like hip fractures and metabolic bone disorders. An analysis of the former Yorkshire regional health authority's hospital activity statistics shows that age-adjusted rates for these opportunistic diagnoses are greater than expected for older people. This indicates substantial 'hidden' alcohol-related morbidity in people aged 65 years and over.

People with learning difficulties rarely get included in discussions of alcohol-related problems. In the past, the practice of institutionalisation meant that many people with learning difficulties never had access to alcohol, but as Jill Manthorpe argues in Chapter 4, the principle of normalisation involves the acceptance of greater risks for vulnerable people. If we include people with learning difficulties in social activities which involve alcohol consumption we have to find ways to protect them from alcohol-related harm, and she shows how this is being managed in several localities.

In Chapter 5, Larry Harrison and Hugo Luck examine the prevalence of drinking problems among homeless people in the UK. They review the literature on the nature and meaning of the link between tenure and alcohol dependence, and outline some recent developments involving case management, outreach, and specialised accommodation. Harrison and Luck contend that the disadvantaged are more likely to suffer alcohol-related

problems, even when drinking at the same levels as more
privileged groups, because they lack the material resources, and
often the social supports, available to others.

Roger Marshall demonstrates in Chapter 6 that social factors
like poverty and homelessness are important influences on treatment outcomes. He reviews the research evidence on 'spontaneous
remission', and from treatment evaluation and longitudinal
studies, and suggests that by gaining a better understanding of the
factors which seem to facilitate the process of restitution we will
be able to develop a framework of care for problem drinkers in
the community.

This emphasis on the social and cultural contexts within which
problem drinking takes place, and on the significance of socioeconomic disadvantage, leads on to a consideration of the
particular difficulties faced by women. In Chapter 7, Jan Waterson
presents a critique of views of women's drinking problems which
give primacy to foetal harm, or focus on the deviant status of
female drinkers. She offers an alternative view, which stresses the
importance of gender and socioeconomic position. This is based
on empirical data, drawn from a study of sixty female alcohol
users who did not have identified problems, and who had recently
become mothers for the first time. She argues that conventional
interpretations not only ignore the 'gendering' of alcohol as a
social problem, but also discount the vital importance of social
advantage or disadvantage in both structuring the opportunities
to drink and in creating stresses which might encourage drinking.

This is followed, in Chapter 8, by an evaluation of the research
evidence for the influence of gender on treatment entry and
outcome. Betsy Thom and Anna Green note the poverty of
research on women's use of treatment services – which makes it
difficult to draw firm conclusions which could assist policy-makers
or service providers. Nevertheless, they find widespread agreement regarding some of the factors which appear to influence
women's help-seeking behaviour, and the authors consider the
need for specialist women's services and for gender-sensitive treatment approaches.

Chapter 9 continues the theme of removing barriers to service
access, but in relation to Black communities in the UK.
Larry Harrison, Mary Harrison and Victor Adebowale review the
existing epidemiological evidence on the prevalence of drinking
problems among Black people, before recent data on mortality

by country of birth are considered. These data indicate that the conventional view – that there are low levels of drinking problems among African–Caribbean men – may have to be revised. In the light of these findings, and evidence that racism, often operating at a covert level, discourages Black people from seeking help, the authors discuss how treatment services could improve access for ethnic minorities.

Chapter 10 examines the implications of recent British community-care legislation for alcohol services. Larry Harrison, Philip Guy and Wayne Sivyer trace the post-war development of alcohol treatment services before considering how the present pattern of provision will be affected by the introduction of a purchaser–provider split. As a case study, they take two local authorities and show how the implementation of the government's community-care policy led to the temporary loss of direct services, a rise in administration costs, and conflict between social services, probation and the non-statutory sector. The authors record how growing pressures for cost-effectiveness are likely to reduce reliance on residential rehabilitation. Finally, they assess how changes in the health policy process might influence the future development of alcohol services.

REFERENCES

Abel, P. (1983) *Alcohol Related Problems in Social Work Caseloads*, Bristol: Social Services Department, Avon County Council.

Alaszewski, A. and Harrison, L. (1992) 'Alcohol and social work: a literature review', *British Journal of Social Work*, 22(3): 331–43.

Bien, T. H., Miller, W. R. and Tonigan, J. S. (1993) 'Brief interventions for alcohol problems: a review', *Addiction*, 88(3): 315–36.

Brown, G. W. and Harris, T. O. (1978) *Social Origins of Depression*, London: Tavistock.

Bruun, K., Lumio, M., Mèkela, K., Pan, L., Popham, R., Room, R., Schmidt, W., Skog, O., Sulkunnen, P. and Osterberg, E. (1975) *Alcohol Control Policies in Public Health Perspective*, Helsinki: Finnish Foundation for Alcohol Studies.

Cahalan, D. and Room, R. (1974) *Problem Drinking Among American Men*, New Brunswick, NJ: Rutgers University.

Cloninger, C. R., Bohan, M. and Sigvardsson, S. (1981) 'Inheritance of alcohol abuse: cross-fostering analysis of adopted men', *Archives of General Psychiatry*, 38: 861–8.

Cochrane, R. (1983) *The Social Creation of Mental Illness*, Harlow: Longman.

Cochrane, R. and Stopes-Roe, M. (1980) 'Factors effecting the distribution of psychological symptoms in urban areas of England', *Acta Psychiatrica Scandinavica*, 61: 445–60.

Davidson, R., Rollnick, S. and MacEwan, I., (eds) (1991) *Counselling Problem Drinkers*, London: Routledge & Kegan Paul.

Department of Health and Social Security (1981) *Prevention and Health: Drinking Sensibly*, London: HMSO.

Department of Health and Social Security and the Welsh Office (1978) *The Pattern and Range of Services for Problem Drinkers: Report of the Advisory Committee on Alcoholism*, London: HMSO.

Edwards, G., Anderson, G., Anderson, P., Babor, T. F., Casswell, S., Ferrence, R., Giesbrecht, N., Godfrey, C., Holder, H. D., Lemmens, P., Makela, K., Midanik, L. T., Norstrom, T., Osterberg, E., Romelsjo, A., Room, R., Simpura, J. and Skog, O. (1994) *Alcohol Policy and the Public Good*, Oxford: Oxford University Press.

Gallup, G. H. (1976) *Gallup International Opinion Polls, Great Britain, 1937–75*, New York: Random House.

Glass, I. B. (1989) 'Undergraduate medical training in substance abuse in the United Kingdom', *British Journal of Addiction*, 84(2): 197–202.

Goddard, E. and Ikin, C. (1988) *Drinking in England and Wales in 1987*, London: HMSO.

Godfrey, C. and Harrison, L. (1990) 'Preventive health objectives and tax policy options', in A. Maynard and P. Tether (eds) *The Addiction Market: Consumption, Production and Policy Development*, Aldershot: Avebury.

Goldberg, D. and Huxley, P. (1992) *Common Mental Disorders: a Biosocial Model*, London: Tavistock/Routledge.

Graham, H. (1993) *When Life's a Drag: Women, Smoking and Disadvantage*, London: HMSO.

Harrison, L. (1989) 'The information component', in D. Robinson, A. Maynard and R. Chester (eds) *Controlling Legal Addictions*, London: Macmillan.

Harrison, L. (1992a) 'Substance misuse and social work qualifying training in the British Isles: a survey of CQSW courses', *British Journal of Addiction*, 87(4): 635–42.

Harrison, L. (ed.) (1992b) *Substance Misuse: Guidance Notes for the Diploma in Social Work*, Improving Social Work Education and Training 14, London: Central Council for Education and Training in Social Work.

Harrison, L. (1993a) *Alcohol Problems: A Resource Directory and Bibliography*, London: Central Council for Education and Training in Social Work.

Harrison, L., (ed.) (1993b) *Substance Misuse: Designing Social Work Training*, London: Central Council for Education and Training in Social Work.

Harrison, L., Carr-Hill, R. and Sutton, M. (1993) 'Consumption and harm: drinking patterns of the Irish, the English and the Irish in England', *Alcohol and Alcoholism*, 28(6): 715–23.

Heather, N. (1987) 'DRAMS for problem drinkers: the potential of a brief intervention by general practitioners and some evidence of its effectiveness', in T. Stockwell and S. Clement (eds) *Helping the Problem Drinker: New Initiatives in Community Care*, London: Croom Helm.

Heather, N. (1994) 'Brief interventions on the world map', *Addiction*, 89(6): 665–7.

Heather, N. and Robertson, I. (1983) *Controlled Drinking*, London: Methuen.

Hodgson, R. (1989) 'Low cost responses', in D. Robinson, A. Maynard and R. Chester (eds) *Controlling Legal Addictions*, London: Macmillan.

Jarman, C. and Kellett, J. (1979) 'Alcoholism in the general hospital', *British Medical Journal*, 2: 469–72.

Levin, J. D. (1990) *Alcoholism: A Bio-psycho-social Approach*, London: Hemisphere Publications.

Lewis, D. C. (1989) 'Putting training about alcohol and other drugs into the mainstream of medical education', *Alcohol Health and Research World*, 13: 8–14.

Marsh, A. and McKay, S. (1994) *Poor Smokers*, London: Policy Studies Institute.

Miller, W. R. (1983) 'Controlled drinking: a history and a critical review', *Journal of Studies on Alcohol*, 44(1): 68–83.

Miller, W. R. (1992) 'The effectiveness of treatment for substance abuse: reasons for optimism', *Journal of Substance Abuse Treatment*, 9(2): 93–102.

Miller, B. A., Downs, W. R. and Testa, M. (1993) 'Interrelationships between victimisation experiences and women's alcohol/drug use', *Journal of Studies in Alcohol*, (suppl) 11: 109–17.

Miller, W. and Rollnick, S., (eds) (1991) *Motivational Interviewing: Preparing People to Change Addictive Behaviors*, New York: Guilford Press.

National Opinion Polls (1984) *Political, Social and Economic Review*, London: National Opinion Polls Market Research Ltd.

Pearson, G. (1987) *The New Heroin Users*, London: Blackwell.

Prochaska, J. and DiClemente, C. (1986) 'Toward a comprehensive model of change', in W. R. Miller and H. Heather (eds) *Treating Addictive Behaviours*, New York, NY: Plenum Press.

Robinson, D., Tether, P. and Teller, J., (eds) (1989) *Local Action on Alcohol Problems*, London: Tavistock/Routledge.

Rollnick, S. (1985) 'The value of a cognitive-behavioural approach in the treatment of problem drinkers', in N. Heather, I. Robertson and P. Davies (eds) *The Misuse of Alcohol: Crucial Issues in Dependence, Treatment and Prevention*, London: Croom Helm.

Rollnick, S., Heather, N. and Bell, A. (1992) 'Negotiating behaviour change in medical settings: the development of brief motivational interviewing', *Journal of Mental Health*, 1: 25–37.

Room, R. (1977) 'The measurement and distribution of drinking patterns and problems in general populations', in G. Edwards, M. Gross, M. Keller, J. Moser and R. Room (eds) *Alcohol Related Disabilities*,

Geneva: World Health Organisation.

Royal College of Psychiatrists (1979) *Alcohol and Alcoholism*, London: Tavistock.

Sanchez-Craig, M., Annia, H. M., Bornet, A. R. and MacDonald, K. R. (1984) 'Random assignment to abstinence and controlled drinking: evaluation of a cognitive-behavioural program for problem drinkers', *Journal of Consulting and Clinical Psychology*, 52(3): 390–403.

Scottish Office (1993) *Towards a National Strategy for Substance Misuse in Scotland*, Edinburgh: HMSO.

Shaw, S., Cartwright, A., Spratley, T. and Harwin, J. (1978) *Responding to Drinking Problems*, London: Croom Helm.

Spratley, T. A., Cartwright, A. K. J. and Shaw, S. J. (1977) 'Alcoholism: the changing role of the psychiatrist', in G. Edwards and M. Grant (eds) *Alcoholism: New Knowledge and New Responses*, London: Croom Helm.

Tether, P. and Robinson, D. (1986) *Preventing Alcohol Problems: a Guide to Local Action*, London: Tavistock.

Townsend, P. and Davidson, N., (eds) (1982) *Inequalities in Health: the Black Report*, Harmondsworth: Penguin.

Vaillant, G. (1983) *The Natural History of Alcoholism*, London: Harvard University Press.

Vaillant, G. (1994) 'Evidence that the Type 1/Type 2 dichotomy in alcoholism must be re-examined', *Addiction*, 89(9): 1049–57.

Vaillant, G. and Milofsky, E. (1982) 'Natural history of male alcoholism, IV: paths to recovery', *Archives of General Psychiatry*, 39: 127–31.

Chapter 1

Inter-generational links between childhood abuse and alcohol-related problems

William R. Downs and Brenda A. Miller

INTRODUCTION

Both childhood violence and alcohol problems are widespread in the US. In a nationally representative sample of 6,002 families, Straus and Gelles (1990) found that 11 per cent of children (approximately 6.9 million) were annual victims of parental violence (defined as being hit with an object, kicked, bitten, punched, beat up, burned, scalded, or threatened or attacked with a knife or gun). From 20 to 30 per cent of adult women and from 10 to 15 per cent of adult men report having been sexually abused during childhood (Finkelhor 1979; Finkelhor *et al.* 1989). Williams *et al.* (1989) estimated that 4.6 million women met DSM-III diagnostic criteria, for alcohol abuse or dependence, and estimates of male–female ratios of clinically diagnosable alcohol disorders have ranged from $2:1$ (Williams *et al.* 1989) to $8:1$ (Robins *et al.* 1988). Zucker (1986) estimated an average lifetime diagnosis of alcohol abuse/dependence of 24.3 per cent for men and 4.4 per cent for women, averaged across three Epidemiologic Catchment Area (ECA) sites.

Whether alcohol problems are associated with childhood violence is an important issue both theoretically and clinically. If children whose parents have alcohol problems have an elevated risk of childhood maltreatment, and if childhood maltreatment is then related to the development of alcohol problems for those children in adulthood, then there exists the possibility of inter-generational transmission of both childhood maltreatment and alcohol problems. This chapter examines whether experiences of childhood violence are related to alcohol problems in the parents of the child and whether experiences of childhood violence are related to the development of adulthood alcohol problems for the victims of that violence. Thus, we examine the inter-generational links between parental alcohol problems and childhood violence. In addition, we examine these associations controlling for the gender of the parent with alcohol problems as well as gender of the parent who perpetrates childhood violence. Finally, we examine the literature for these associations as well as report data from a recent study funded by the US National Institute on Alcohol Abuse and Alcoholism (NIAAA).

PARENTAL ALCOHOL PROBLEMS AND CHILDHOOD MALTREATMENT

Literature review

Early reviews of the literature indicated a lack of support for the association between parental alcohol problems and the per-petration of childhood violence by the parents, and severely criticised existing empirical literature for methodological inepti-tude (e.g. Orme and Rimmer 1981). A later review also indicated that the link between parental alcoholism and perpetration of child abuse, if any, may be due to third variables such as socioe-conomic status (SES) (West and Prinz 1987). Other researchers have concluded that only a modest association exists between perpetration of physical child abuse and parental alcohol prob-lems (e.g. Black and Mayer 1980).

More recent and methodologically sophisticated studies, using indices such as the Conflict Tactics Scale and improved sampling techniques, have supported the association between parental alcohol problems and experiences of violence for their children (Kantor and Straus 1990; Radomsky 1991; Famularo et al. 1992a, 1992b; Kantor 1992). In a study of alcoholism in the general population, Holmes and Robins (1988) found parental alcoholism to be related to perpetration of harsh and unfair discipline on the children of the alcoholics. Williams-Petersen et al. (1994) found that drug use is related to child-abuse potential among a prenatal group of women. Reider et al. (1989) found an association between both father's and mother's aggres-sion toward their children and lifetime alcohol problems, controlling for antisocial behaviour, depression, and marital aggression.

In exploring these relationships it is important to distinguish between mother and father violence (Straus *et al.* 1980; Allen and Epperson 1993). Perpetration of childhood violence may be specific to the parent with the alcohol problems. If so, combining both parents in the analysis may attenuate the association between parental alcohol-related problems and childhood maltreatment, or mask gender-related associations. For example, in a sample of male parolees Miller (1990) found that father alcohol problems were related to father-to-parolee but not mother-to-parolee violence, and that mother alcohol problems were related to mother-to-parolee but not father-to-parolee violence, when the parolee was a child.

Yet another issue not addressed systematically in the empirical literature is whether parental alcohol problems are related to experiences of childhood maltreatment from adults outside the nuclear family. This question may be especially poignant for victims of sexual abuse (Miller and Downs 1995). Parental pre-occupation with abusing alcohol or coping with a partner who abuses alcohol may result in neglect of children, which in turn may place these children at risk of other adults who perpetrate sexual abuse on them. Parental unavailability has been found to be associated with childhood sexual abuse (Finkelhor and Baron 1986). In addition, children of alcoholic parents may not experience the nurturing parent-to-child relationship that other children experience, thereby increasing psychological vulnerability to the manipulations of perpetrators who link adult nurturance with sexual access to the child.

In sum, more recent and methodologically sophisticated studies have indicated that parental alcohol problems are related to the perpetration of abuse against their children. However, several issues remain to be addressed by future research. There is a need to control for the gender of the parent with the alcohol problems and perpetrating the violence. Further, there is a need to examine experiences of childhood violence perpetrated by other adults in addition to the parent with the alcohol problems. There is also a need to control for additional variables, such as SES, that may account for the association between parental alcohol problems and experiences of childhood violence. To address these issues, a study concerning the association between family violence and alcohol problems for women and funded by the NIAAA was conducted from 1988–1992.

NIAAA STUDY

Methodology

Samples of women ages 18–45 (N = 472) were recruited from clinical and nonclinical sources in Western New York. The clinical sources consisted of women from outpatient alcoholism clinics (N = 98), women receiving services from shelters or support groups for women experiencing partner violence (N = 97); and women in outpatient mental health clinics (N = 77) (total N = 272). Nonclinical sources included women attending drinking and driving classes following conviction for a driving while intoxicated (DWI) offence – hereafter referred to as the DWI sample (N = 100); and women from households obtained through random digit dialling (N = 100) – hereafter referred to as the community sample (Miller *et al.* 1993; Miller and Downs 1995). The total nonclinical sample size was thus 200.

Women who were currently receiving treatment for alcoholism from one of six clinics in Western New York were recruited at the clinics either through personal contact by one of the interviewers or through flyers which were given to eligible women by their counsellors. The majority of the battered women (77 per cent) were recruited during their stay at a shelter for battered women through personal contact with one of the interviewers during one of the house meetings. The remainder were receiving counselling services for battered women at an agency affiliated with the shelter. They were either given flyers by their counsellors or contacted by an interviewer before the start of their group counselling session.

Women in mental health treatment at six different clinics in Western New York were recruited through flyers which were given to them by their counsellors. Women who were either actively psychotic or suicidally depressed were excluded from the research. In the first instance, actively psychotic women were not expected to be able to provide reliable data for the study. In the second instance, the exclusion was based upon the concern for the women; the interview dealt with extremely sensitive issues and there was concern that the interview process might contribute to negative consequences for the women.

The DWI sample consisted of women who had been arrested for driving while intoxicated and chose to attend a series of seven

drinking driver education classes in order to maintain a condi-
tional licence. Women arrested for DWI who chose to have their
licence suspended or who had been arrested more than once in
the past five years for DWI did not participate in the classes.
One of the interviewers described the study at the end of one
of the classes and offered women the chance to participate.
Although these women experienced an intervention involving
their drinking, they were not seeking treatment and hence are
considered a nonclinical sample.

The community sample was recruited through random digit
dialling in the Buffalo area. If there was a woman in the household between the ages of 18 and 45 the study was described briefly
to her and participation was solicited. Out of a total of 331 contacts
with women aged 18–45, 34 per cent refused before hearing
the description of the study, another 29 per cent refused after
hearing about the study, 7 per cent agreed to be interviewed but
failed to establish or keep appointments, and 30 per cent were
interviewed.

Two in-depth interviews were conducted, with an 18-month time
lag between the first and second interview. A major purpose of
the first interview was to examine associations among parental
alcohol problems, experiences of childhood violence, and development of adulthood alcohol problems for women. Data from this
first interview is reported in the present study. A major purpose
of the second interview was to examine longitudinal associations
between alcohol problems and experiences of partner violence for
women. This data is reported elsewhere (e.g. Downs and Miller
1994). Each participant completed a two and a half hour, face-to-
face, in-depth interview that included both structured and
open-ended questions. Prior to signing informed consents, participants were told that the interview would include questions about
childhood family relationships, childhood sexual experiences,
parental alcohol and drug use, current family, relationship with
spouse/partner, and her own and her partner's alcohol and drug
use. All respondents were asked and agreed to allow audio taping
of the interview.

Measures

This research utilised in-depth face-to-face interviews to assess
multiple types of childhood victimisation. Multiple questions were

used to assess childhood sexual abuse, and mother and father verbal, moderate and severe violence. Measures of childhood sexual abuse included experiences that occurred prior to 18 years of age for the woman. A list of childhood sexual abuse incidents defined by Finkelhor (1979), and supplemented by items from Sgroi (1982), was used to generate a list of sexual abuse experiences for girls. These experiences included:

- invitation or suggestion to do something sexual;
- other person showing his/her genitals to you, you showing your genitals to another person;
- kissing or hugging in a sexual way;
- other person fondling you in a sexual way;
- you fondling other person in a sexual way;
- other person touching your genitals either with his/her hands or mouth;
- you touching other person's genitals either with your hands or mouth;
- person rubbing his/her genitals on your body without penetration;
- intercourse;
- other person putting finger into your vagina or anus.

(Miller *et al.* 1993)

Sexual abuse was then defined as follows:

victimisation experiences prior to the age of 18 and that occurred against the victim's will or under conditions that would not allow the victim to consent with full knowledge.

This definition follows guidelines established by Finkelhor (1979). Perpetrators included any relative, someone at least five years older than the victim, or anyone who forced sexual activity against the victim's will. To limit the measure to the most potentially harmful sexual experiences, we excluded any boyfriend experience that was defined as consensual by the woman, even if the boyfriend was more than five years older.

Parental violence was assessed by indices based on the Conflict Tactics Scale or CTS (Straus 1979; Straus *et al.* 1980). Measures of both mother-to-daughter violence and father-to-daughter violence were included. If more than one mother and/or father figure were present during the woman's childhood, the parental figure that was predominant (longest duration) was used in these analyses. The CTS measures negative verbal interaction, moderate physical violence, and severe physical violence. The CTS was modified slightly for the present study. Two items were added to the negative verbal interaction index: 'insulted or swore at you in a sexual manner' and 'threatened to abandon you.'

For the present analysis, verbal aggression was conceptualised as the independent variable, instead of negative verbal interaction. Thus, three items ('sulk and/or refuse to talk about it'; 'stomp out of the room or house'; 'cry') were excluded from the present analysis. Second, because virtually all respondents stated that their mothers and fathers had slapped or spanked them, this item was excluded from the analysis for the moderate violence scale.

The modified CTS used in the study consisted of four verbal aggression items, four moderate violence items, and seven severe violence items. Each item on the CTS sub-scales was dichotomised into 0 = never happened and 1 = happened at least once. One point was scored for each item that happened at least once and points were summed across items for each sub-scale. Thus the range for the verbal aggression and moderate violence sub-scales was 0–4, and for severe violence was 0–7. This measure provided an index of the number or range of different items each respondent experienced for each sub-scale. Respondents reported separate CTS sub-scale scores for mother-to-daughter and father-to-daughter interactions during childhood. For brevity, these scores are referred to as 'mother' and 'father' scores, respectively.

In addition, the number of items experienced from either parent was calculated and referred to as the 'parent' score. There were also assessments of parental alcohol problems for both father and mother; number of changes in the family structure (e.g., divorces, death); socioeconomic status of the family in childhood; and race of respondent. Women were given self-administered forms assessing parental alcohol and drug problems based on criteria derived from the Research Diagnostic Criteria (RDC) (Andreasen et al. 1977). Three variables were created based on the RDC criteria: father alcohol problems, mother alcohol problems, and parental alcohol problems. Socioeconomic status for the respondent's family of origin was calculated using the Hollingshead index. A series of items assessed number of changes in childhood family structure (e.g., parental divorce, parental separation, death in the family). Multiple occurrences of the same change were counted as additional changes. These items were then summed to provide an index for the number of changes in childhood family structure.

RESULTS

Parental alcohol problems and childhood maltreatment

A two-way analysis of covariance (ANCOVA) was performed with type of sample as one independent variable, and parental, father, or mother alcohol problems as the second independent variable. Covariates included race of respondent, number of changes in childhood family structure, and childhood SES. Covariates were entered first in all analyses. The interaction effect between the independent variables was also tested. Dependent variables examined sequentially included father violence, mother violence, and childhood sexual abuse.

The ANCOVAs for the associations between parental alcohol problems and each form of childhood violence were performed first. The association between parental alcohol problems and father violence was significantly different from zero (F = 16.032, p < 0.000). Respondents with at least one parent who has an alcohol problem reported a significantly higher level of father violence than respondents with neither parent having an alcohol problem. Also, the association between parental alcohol problems and childhood sexual abuse was significantly different from zero (F = 7.303, p = 0.007).

Respondents with at least one parent who has an alcohol problem were significantly more likely to report sexual abuse than respondents with neither parent reporting an alcohol problem. However, the association between parental alcohol problems and mother violence was not significantly different from zero (F = 1.437, p = 0.231). The ANCOVAs for the associations between father alcohol problems and each form of childhood violence were performed next, and are reported in Tables 1.1–1.3.

An interesting pattern begins to appear in the data. The main effects for father alcohol problems in predicting father violence (see Table 1.1) and childhood sexual abuse (Table 1.3) were statistically different from zero. Presence of father alcohol problems was related to greater levels of father violence and increased likelihood of sexual abuse compared with absence of father

Table 1.1 Father-to-daughter severe violence by father's alcohol problems and type of sample, controlling for race, SES, and changes in childhood family structure (mean scores)

		FATHER'S ALCOHOL PROBLEMS	
		No	*Yes*
TYPE OF SAMPLE	*Non-clinical*	0.15 (131)	0.55 (58)
	Clinical	0.47 (137)	1.24 (116)

Source of variation	Sum of squares	DF	Mean square	F	Sig of F
COVARIATES	22.149	3	7.383	5.977	0.001
Race	1.952	1	1.952	1.580	0.209
Changes in childhood family	10.848	1	10.848	8.782	0.003
Childhood SES	9.898	1	9.898	8.013	0.005
MAIN EFFECTS	58.264	2	29.132	23.584	0.000
Type of sample	16.696	1	16.696	13.516	0.000
Father alcohol problems	35.138	1	35.138	28.446	0.000
2-WAY INTERACTIONS Type of sample Father alcohol problems	3.317	1	3.317	2.685	0.102
Explained	83.729	6	13.955	11.297	0.000
Residual	537.330	435	1.235		
Total	621.059	441	1.408		

COVARIATE RAW REGRESSION COEFFICIENT	
Race	0.164
Changes in childhood family	0.082
Childhood SES	−0.012

alcohol problems. However, the main effect for father alcohol problems in predicting mother violence (Table 1.2) was not statistically different from zero. Finally, the ANCOVAs for the associations between mother alcohol problems and each form of childhood violence are reported in Tables 1.4–1.6.

Another interesting pattern appears in the data. The main effects for mother alcohol problems in predicting father violence (Table 1.4) and childhood sexual abuse (Table 1.6) were not statis-

Table 1.2 Mother-to-daughter severe violence by father's alcohol problems and type of sample, controlling for race, SES, and changes in childhood family structure (mean scores)

		FATHER'S ALCOHOL PROBLEMS	
		No	Yes
TYPE OF SAMPLE	Non-clinical	0.37 (131)	0.59 (58)
	Clinical	1.05 (137)	0.80 (116)

Source of variation	Sum of squares	DF	Mean square	F	Sig of F
COVARIATES	58.727	3	19.576	15.095	0.000
Race	2.066	1	2.066	1.593	0.208
Changes in childhood family	39.014	1	39.014	30.085	0.000
Childhood SES	2.277	1	2.277	1.756	0.186
MAIN EFFECTS	9.919	2	4.959	3.824	0.023
Type of sample	9.055	1	9.055	6.982	0.009
Father alcohol problems	1.622	1	1.622	1.251	0.264
2-WAY INTERACTIONS	3.571	1	3.571	2.754	0.098
Type of sample Father alcohol problems					
Explained	72.216	6	12.036	9.281	0.000
Residual	564.110	435	1.297		
Total	636.326	441	1.443		

COVARIATE RAW REGRESSION COEFFICIENT
Race   −0.168
Changes in childhood family   0.155
Childhood SES   −0.006

tically different from zero. However, the main effect for mother alcohol problems in predicting mother violence was statistically different from zero (see Table 1.5). Presence of mother alcohol problems was related to greater levels of mother violence. In all ANCOVAs, the main effect for type of sample was statistically significant, with clinical sample respondents reporting higher levels of the childhood violence variable being tested than did the non-clinical sample respondents, with the exception of Table 1.5.

Table 1.3   Childhood sexual abuse by father's alcohol problems and type of sample, controlling for race, SES, and changes in childhood family structure (mean scores)

		FATHER'S ALCOHOL PROBLEMS	
		No	Yes
TYPE OF SAMPLE	*Non-clinical*	0.25 (131)	0.43 (58)
	Clinical	0.58 (137)	0.72 (116)

Source of variation	Sum of squares	DF	Mean square	F	Sig of F
COVARIATES	6.368	3	2.123	9.925	0.000
Race	0.121	1	0.121	0.565	0.453
Changes in childhood family	4.896	1	4.896	22.893	0.000
Childhood SES	0.858	1	0.858	4.012	0.046
MAIN EFFECTS	11.066	2	5.533	25.869	0.000
Type of sample	8.023	1	8.023	37.514	0.000
Father alcohol problems	1.967	1	1.967	9.198	0.003
2-WAY INTERACTIONS Type of sample Father alcohol problems	0.026	1	0.026	0.121	0.728
Explained	17.460	6	2.910	13.606	0.000
Residual	93.038	435	0.214		
Total	110.498	441	0.251		

COVARIATE RAW REGRESSION COEFFICIENT	
Race	0.041
Changes in childhood family	0.055
Childhood SES	−0.004

The interaction effect examines whether the relationship between parental alcohol problems and childhood violence differs across the two sample types. None of these interaction effects were statistically significant, indicating that the relationship between parental alcohol problems and each form of childhood violence did not differ in the clinical sample as compared with the non-clinical sample. The covariates did differ in their associations with the different forms of childhood violence however.

Table 1.4   Father-to-daughter severe violence by mother's alcohol problems and type of sample, controlling for race, SES, and changes in childhood family structure (mean scores)

		MOTHER'S ALCOHOL PROBLEMS	
		No	Yes
TYPE OF SAMPLE	Non-clinical	0.28 (174)	0.20 (15)
	Clinical	0.87 (198)	0.65 (55)

Source of variation	Sum of squares	DF	Mean square	F	Sig of F
COVARIATES	22.149	3	7.383	5.607	0.001
Race	1.952	1	1.952	1.483	0.224
Changes in childhood family	10.848	1	10.848	8.239	0.004
Childhood SES	9.898	1	9.898	7.517	0.006
MAIN EFFECTS	25.904	2	12.952	9.836	0.000
Type of sample	25.082	1	25.082	19.049	0.000
Mother alcohol problems	2.778	1	2.778	2.110	0.147
2-WAY INTERACTIONS Type of sample Mother alcohol problems	0.216	1	0.216	0.164	0.686
Explained	48.269	6	8.045	6.110	0.000
Residual	572.790	435	1.317		
Total	621.059	441	1.408		

COVARIATE RAW REGRESSION COEFFICIENT
Race   0.164
Changes in childhood family   0.082
Childhood SES   −0.012

Number of changes in childhood family and childhood SES were significant predictors of father violence. A greater number of childhood family changes and a lower childhood SES were associated with higher levels of father violence. Only number of changes in childhood family predicted mother violence. A greater number of childhood family changes was associated with a higher level of mother violence. Finally, number of changes in childhood family and childhood SES were significant predictors of childhood sexual

Table 1.5 Mother-to-daughter severe violence by mother's alcohol problems and type of sample, controlling for race, SES, and changes in childhood family structure (mean scores)

		MOTHER'S ALCOHOL PROBLEMS	
		No	*Yes*
TYPE OF SAMPLE	*Non-clinical*	0.39 (174)	1.00 (15)
	Clinical	0.75 (198)	1.60 (55)

Source of variation	Sum of squares	DF	Mean square	F	Sig of F
COVARIATES	58.727	3	19.576	15.698	0.000
Race	2.066	1	2.066	1.657	0.199
Changes in childhood family	39.014	1	39.014	31.287	0.000
Childhood SES	2.277	1	2.277	1.826	0.177
MAIN EFFECTS	35.022	2	17.511	14.043	0.000
Type of sample	4.203	1	4.203	3.371	0.067
Mother alcohol problems	26.725	1	26.725	21.432	0.000
2-WAY INTERACTIONS Type of sample Mother alcohol problems	0.139	1	0.139	0.111	0.739
Explained	93.887	6	15.648	12.549	0.000
Residual	542.439	435	1.247		
Total	636.326	441	1.443		

COVARIATE	RAW REGRESSION COEFFICIENT
Race	−0.168
Changes in childhood family	0.155
Childhood SES	−0.006

abuse. A greater number of childhood family changes and a lower childhood SES were associated with a higher likelihood of sexual abuse having occurred. Race of respondent was unrelated to any of the forms of childhood violence.

Table 1.6 Childhood sexual abuse by mother's alcohol problems
and type of sample, controlling for race, SES, and
changes in childhood family structure (mean scores)

		MOTHER'S ALCOHOL PROBLEMS	
		No	Yes
TYPE OF SAMPLE	Non-clinical	0.30 (174)	0.40 (15)
	Clinical	0.63 (198)	0.73 (55)

Source of variation	Sum of squares	DF	Mean square	F	Sig of F
COVARIATES	6.3687	3	2.123	9.7458	0.000
Race	0.121	1	0.121	0.555	0.457
Changes in childhood family	4.896	1	4.896	22.478	0.000
Childhood SES	0.858	1	0.858	3.940	0.048
MAIN EFFECTS	9.372	2	4.686	21.512	0.000
Type of sample	8.410	1	8.410	38.608	0.000
Mother alcohol problems	0.273	1	0.273	1.254	0.263
2-WAY INTERACTIONS	0.003	1	0.003	0.012	0.913
Type of sample Father alcohol problems					
Explained	15.743	6	2.624	12.045	0.000
Residual	94.755	435	0.218		
Total	110.498	441	0.251		

COVARIATE RAW REGRESSION COEFFICIENT
Race   0.041
Changes in childhood family   0.055
Childhood SES   −0.004

Physical abuse and parental alcohol problems

Thus, for parental severe violence, alcohol problems were related
to greater levels of childhood violence for the parent with those
alcohol problems. However, alcohol problems in one parent were
not related to greater levels of violence in the other parent. These
findings are identical to those of Miller (1990) who found that
father alcohol problems were related to father but not mother

violence, and that mother alcohol problems were related to mother but not father violence. \|

Furthermore, these findings demonstrate the need to examine these associations specifically for the gender of the parent regarding their alcohol problems and perpetration of violence. Had we not done so, we would have been left with the conclusion simply that parental alcohol problems are associated with father violence but not mother violence. These results indicate that severe violence against children is directly related to the alcohol problems of the perpetrator of the violence.

However, the cross-sectional nature of the present study precludes any conclusions concerning causal pathways between parental alcohol problems and childhood violence. It is possible that parents may develop alcohol problems as a function of per- petrating severe violence against their children. For example, parents may feel guilty as a result of observing the effect of this violence on their children. This set of dynamics would be similar to the development of alcohol problems secondary to the initial development of depression. However, the bio-psycho-social matrix in which alcohol problems are presumed to develop makes this causal pathway unlikely. For example, findings from the Epi- demiologic Catchment Area (ECA) study indicated that a large majority of men with co-existing depression and alcohol problems experience secondary depression, that is depression whose onset follows that of the chronic alcohol abuse (Helzer and Pryzbeck 1988) as opposed to preceding it. In other words, it is more likely that the parent's alcohol problems are derived from other causes and result in severe violence against children rather than the reverse.

The results of the present study do not clarify how parental alcohol problems may result in the perpetration of severe violence against their children. Various hypotheses have been proposed to account for the link between alcohol use and violence. First, the disinhibition hypothesis posits a direct pharmacological link between alcohol use and aggression and thus is largely physio- logical in nature. This hypothesis has received little empirical support however (Pernanen 1981; White 1990; Fagan 1993).

Second, according to the cognitive disorganisation hypothesis, alcohol use alters perception of environmental cues, typically resulting in an over-estimation of environmental threat, and an increased likelihood of violence (Richardson 1981). While drinking, already stressed individuals may misinterpret inter-personal cues and be more likely to resort to violence than other individuals. In a related theoretical development, Steele and Josephs (1990) have theorised that alcohol makes social behaviours more extreme by blocking the conflicting response. There is very little data regarding the cognitive disorganisation hypothesis, however.

Third, in the deviance disavowal/expectancy hypothesis, drinking allows the perpetrator to 'construct a story' that acknowledges the violence but allows him or her to continue to believe that it is 'normal' by attributing the violence to the use of alcohol. Thus, alcohol does not act pharmacologically to increase violence but, due to cultural expectancies about the effects of alcohol, functions as a rationale for violence. Thus, inter-personal violence is contextualised, and is a function of the alcohol itself, the physical setting of use, norms about violence in that setting, and cultural expectations about violence (Fagan 1993).

Fourth, Kantor and Straus (1990) found parents with the highest levels of abuse to be mothers with binge drinking patterns and fathers with high daily alcohol consumption patterns. Thus, pattern of drinking may be a contributing factor to parental violence. Further, pattern of alcohol use may interact with gender of the perpetrating parent in complex ways to result in perpetration of physical abuse against their children. Alternatively, the association between parental alcohol problems and childhood violence may be spurious and due to their common associations with a third factor uncontrolled for in the present study.

One such factor could be anti-social personality disorder. Anti-social personality disorder has been found to be related to the early onset of alcohol problems, referred to as primary ASP and secondary alcoholism (Schuckit 1973; Hesselbrock et al. 1985; Liskow et al. 1991); Type II alcoholism (Cloninger 1987); or as Type B alcoholism (Babor et al. 1992). Also, DiLalla and Gottesman (1991) suggested that children of ASP-positive parents are more likely to be physically abused than children of ASP-negative parents.

However, there are serious empirical and definitional problems with this line of theoretical work. First, ASP disorder can only account for a minority of alcohol problems. Helzer and Pryzbeck (1988) found only a 15 per cent prevalence rate of ASP disorder among alcoholics in the Epidemiologic Catchment Area (ECA) study. Further, Alterman and Cacciola (1991) have noted some problems with the ASP disorder diagnosis itself, including low inter-rater reliability and low diagnostic stability – in part because the operationalisation of criteria are related to the referential frameworks of those making the assessments. Instead of the psychiatric diagnosis of ASP disorder as an explanatory variable, criminal behaviour in general may be related to both parental alcohol problems and perpetration of childhood maltreatment, with all three problems arising in the context of deprived environments. More research is needed to unravel additional factors that may be related to both parental alcohol problems and childhood maltreatment.

In sum, recent data from a large study funded by the NIAAA has indicated that parental alcohol problems are related to the perpetration of physical violence specifically by the parent with the alcohol problem. However, alcohol problems in one parent were not found to be related to greater levels of violence in the other parent. Finally, the theoretical links between parental alcohol problems and childhood physical abuse remain unclear.

Sexual abuse and parental alcohol problems

Father alcohol problems were found to be related to experiences of sexual abuse in the present study. However, mother alcohol problems were not found to be related to experiences of childhood sexual abuse. This last result is contrary to previous literature which found mother's drinking to be related to experiences of sexual abuse for daughters (e.g., Finkelhor 1979). For a closer examination of these associations, it is necessary to explore the identity of the sexual abuse perpetrator.

Most of the childhood sexual abuse experiences reported in the NIAAA study were perpetrated by men. Only 3 per cent of the women reported a female perpetrator. However, only 4 per cent of the women reported either a biological or adoptive father as the sexual abuse perpetrator (Miller and Downs 1995). Thus, it is unlikely that the father with the alcohol problems was the perpetrator of the sexual abuse. Instead, others outside the conjugal family are more likely to be the perpetrators of the sexual abuse, although that abuse is more likely to occur in families in which the father has an alcohol problem. These other perpetrators were most likely to be an adult male relative or family friend. A significantly higher percentage of women in the alcoholism treatment sample reported sexual abuse or molestation by any male relative (40 per cent) than women in either the DWI or community samples (9 per cent and 13 per cent respectively) (ibid.). Also, a significantly higher percentage of the women in the alcoholism treatment sample reported a male family friend as a perpetrator (37 per cent) compared with either the DWI (12 per cent) or community samples (16 per cent) (ibid.). Only 9 per cent reported a stranger as a perpetrator of childhood sexual abuse (ibid.).

Previously, a mother's drinking was presumed to increase the likelihood of sexual abuse via her inability to protect daughters from others (e.g. Finkelhor 1979) – including fathers. Lack of maternal protection was presumed to be a function in part of her heavy drinking. In the present work, however, mother alcohol problems were not related to likelihood of sexual abuse experiences. Instead, lack of paternal protection, due to father's alcohol problems, may contribute to other males known to the family perpetrating sexual abuse against daughters.

There are two possible mechanisms by which father alcohol problems may be related to other adult males perpetrating sexual abuse on the daughter. First, daughters growing up in homes with an alcoholic father may not receive the typical emotional support, nurturance, and sustenance from their fathers. As a result, these girls may be more vulnerable to the manipulations of adult males outside the nuclear family who provide that support and nurturance, but at the cost of sexually abusing the girl. Second, daughters in homes with an alcoholic father may be more likely to be placed temporarily with relatives as the parents attempt to cope with the problems of alcohol dependence. These girls may then be more likely to be abused at the homes of these relatives. Additional research is needed to clarify these issues.

CHILDHOOD MALTREATMENT AND THE DEVELOPMENT OF ADULTHOOD ALCOHOL PROBLEMS

Literature review

Recently there has been some controversy regarding whether experiences of childhood violence are in fact related to the development of alcohol problems in adulthood. Research has indicated a weaker link for childhood violence and adolescent alcohol problems than for childhood violence and adulthood alcohol problems. Also, prospective and retrospective research have yielded contradictory results with regard to this association.

In fact, method variance may account for many of the discrepant findings in this area. Wyatt and Peters (1986) found that face-to-face interviews using specific multiple questions resulted in greater rates of reported sexual abuse. Further, Lanktree *et al.* (1991) found that use of medical charts resulted in much lower rates of reported sexual abuse than asking about that abuse. Thus, the associations between experiences of childhood violence and the development of adulthood alcohol problems are complex, and may depend on the gender and developmental stage of the victim as well as the methodology employed in the research.

Adolescents

Research conducted with adolescents has yielded inconsistent findings on the relationship between childhood victimisation and alcohol abuse (e.g. Goldston *et al.* 1989; Harrison *et al.* 1989a, 1989b). However, these studies may have under-identified victims by not using the multiple question technique recommended by Wyatt and Peters (1986). Research by Dembo and colleagues, using a multiple question format and multivariate analysis, has also yielded contradictory findings. Experiences of physical abuse and sexual abuse in childhood had a direct effect on illicit drug use for both males and females (Dembo *et al.* 1987; Dembo *et al.* 1988a, 1988b). However, no association was found between experiences of childhood sexual abuse and alcohol use or between experiences of physical abuse and alcohol use for either males or females (Dembo *et al.* 1988a). Later, Dembo and colleagues (1989) found that physical abuse (but not sexual abuse) was related to alcohol use cross-sectionally but not longitudinally. However, sexual abuse was found to be related to marijuana use longitudinally, and physical abuse was found related to cocaine use longitudinally (Dembo *et al.* 1989).

Further, while Ireland and Widom (1994) found that a history of childhood maltreatment was related to juvenile arrest in general, they did not find that history of childhood maltreatment predicted juvenile arrest specifically for alcohol or drug offences. However, in a recent review of the literature on reported victims of sexual abuse during childhood, Kendall-Tackett *et al.* (1993) reported that approximately 53 per cent of sexually abused adolescents reported substance abuse – a percentage greater than most community studies of sexual abuse.

Adults

Research on adults has also produced some contradictory results. Prospective research typically has not shown a link between experiences of childhood violence and adulthood alcohol problems. Conversely, retrospective research strongly supports the association between experiences of childhood violence and the development of alcohol problems (e.g. Downs *et al.* 1992; Miller and Downs 1993; Miller *et al.* 1993; Miller and Downs 1995).

Reporting the results of a meticulous longitudinal study, McCord (1983) found that parentally abused or neglected males did not differ reliably from parentally loved males in the proportion who became alcoholic in adulthood. History of physical abuse or sexual abuse during childhood did not predict number of lifetime symptoms of alcohol problems, diagnosis of alcohol dependence for men or women, nor arrest for adulthood alcohol or drug offences for men (Ireland and Widom 1994; Widom *et al.* in 1995). Conversely, history of childhood maltreatment was found to be related to arrest for adulthood alcohol or drug offences for women (Ireland and Widom 1994).

However, the past two studies may have under-estimated the effect of childhood maltreatment, since an unknown but large percentage of cases in the non-abused control group may have in fact experienced maltreatment during childhood. Retrospective research has typically demonstrated a link between experiences of childhood violence and the development of alcohol problems in adulthood for both male and female respondents (Rohsenow *et al.* 1988; Hill *et al.* 1992); male respondents (Kroll *et al.* 1985; Holmes and Robins 1987, 1988; Blane *et al.* 1988; Schaefer *et al.* 1988); and female respondents (Covington 1983; Briere and Runtz 1987, 1988; Swett *et al.* 1991).

In a large community survey (N = 3,132 adults), Stein *et al.* (1988) found that history of childhood sexual abuse predicted lifetime diagnosis of drug abuse/dependence – but not alcohol abuse/dependence for men, and both drug abuse/dependence and alcohol abuse for women. Also, using a random sample, Peters

(1988) found childhood sexual abuse to be related to the development of alcohol abuse and other drug abuse for women. Hamberger and Hastings (1987) found that alcoholic batterers were more likely than non-alcoholic batterers to have witnessed father-to-mother violence in childhood.

Differences between mother and father violence

Failure to control for the gender of the parent perpetrating that violence may attenuate the association between experiences of childhood physical violence and the later development of alcohol problems. Allen and Epperson (1993) noted that 'mother-blaming' (the belief that fathers have less influence than mothers on the development of children) has led some researchers to focus on mothers in child maltreatment research. While the rates of mother-to-child serious violence have been found to be higher, potentially lethal forms of violence (e.g. using a knife or gun on the child) were higher for fathers (Straus *et al.* 1980), suggesting that one parent may be more important than the other in understanding the links between experiences of child abuse and the development of adulthood problems in women. Unfortunately, most research has failed to control for gender of the parent in examining these associations.

Prior empirical work by the authors

Starting in 1986, Drs Miller and Downs have investigated the interrelationships among alcohol problems and family violence with a funded pilot project entitled 'Family Violence and Women's Alcohol Use' and subsequently with a previously funded NIAAA study entitled 'The Impact of Family Violence on Women's Alcohol Problems' (1988–92).

In our first study, in-depth interviews were conducted with 45 women who were currently receiving alcoholism treatment or who had received alcoholism treatment previously and were still involved in Alcoholics Anonymous groups in the Western New York area (Downs *et al.* 1987; Miller *et al.* 1987). In addition, 40 women without alcohol problems were drawn from the community using random digit dialling methods to obtain the sample. This first study used measures similar to the later NIAAA study (see pp. 18–21).

Comparisons were made between women alcoholics who had received treatment (N = 45) and women from the community who did not have alcohol problems (N = 40) for rates of father-to-daughter violence, mother-to-daughter violence and childhood sexual abuse (Downs et al. 1987; Miller et al. 1987). Findings revealed that alcoholic women (67 per cent) were 2.5 times more likely to report childhood sexual abuse than non-alcoholic women (28 per cent) (Miller et al. 1987). Alcoholic women also reported approximately twice the levels of father-to-daughter verbal aggression and moderate violence, and approximately four times the level of father-to-daughter severe violence than non-alcoholic women (Downs et al. 1987). The differences in women's experiences of childhood sexual abuse and violence by fathers remained significant, even when parental alcohol problems, number of changes in the family structure, age, and present income source variables – which differed between the two groups – were controlled. Interestingly, there were no significant mother-to-daughter differences in any of the parental violence scales.

However, several questions remained:

1 Can these findings be replicated with a larger sample?
2 Are differences in childhood victimisation rates for alcoholic and non-alcoholic women an artifact of the help-seeking behaviour of alcoholic women?
3 Would other women who are seeking treatment for problems other than alcoholism have similar rates and types of childhood victimisation?
4 Are rates of childhood victimisation greater for women who drink heavily but are not yet alcoholic, or only for women with substantial alcohol problems?

In a subsequent study funded by NIAAA (see pp. 17–27), 472 women were interviewed to examine these questions. The same measures of father and mother violence were used. Sexual abuse experiences were grouped into three categories: invitation, touching, and penetration (Miller et al. 1993).

The first set of comparisons were between women in the alcoholism clinics, DWI, and community samples to determine if the rates of childhood victimisation are higher for all women with heavy drinking patterns or only for women who seek treatment. These results are reported in Table 1.7. In fact, alcoholic women were three times more likely to report being sexually abused as a child (66 per cent) as compared to either the women in the DWI group (21 per cent) or the community group (35 per cent) (Miller *et al.* 1993; Miller and Downs 1995). Furthermore, alcoholic women were significantly more likely to have experienced all three types of sexual abuse (invitation, touching, penetration) as compared to women in the DWI and community samples. For example, alcoholic women were nearly seven times more likely (47 per cent) to experience sexual abuse that involved penetration than the DWI sample (7 per cent) and over five times more likely than the household sample (9 per cent). These differences remained significant when personal and family background characteristics (i.e., race, age, childhood socioeconomic status, parental alcoholism and number of changes in the childhood family structure) were controlled.

Similar results were found for father-to-daughter violence. Alcoholic women were significantly more likely to report father-to-daughter verbal aggression (71 per cent) and severe violence (45 per cent) than either the DWI (verbal 43 per cent, severe 18 per cent) or household groups (verbal 31 per cent, severe 13 per cent) (Miller *et al.* 1993; Miller and Downs 1995). These differences also remained significant when personal characteristics and family background characteristics were controlled. However, while some significant differences were found between groups for levels of mother-to-daughter violence, none of these differences remained significant when personal and family background characteristics were controlled.

To address whether victimisation in childhood has a unique connection to the later development of alcohol problems or is merely an artifact of treatment seeking, women who were in various treatment settings (alcoholism, mental health, and partner violence services) were divided into two groups, consisting of women with (N = 178) and without (N = 92) alcohol problems. These results are reported in Table 1.8. Women in treatment with alcohol problems were significantly more likely to report sexual abuse experiences (70 per cent) than women in treatment without alcohol problems (52 per cent) (Miller *et al.* 1993; Miller and Downs 1995). Moreover, women with alcohol problems were significantly more likely to report both touching and penetration as specific types of sexual abuse. These differences remained significant controlling for parental alcoholism – the only personal

Table 1.7 Percentage experiencing childhood victimisation across alcoholism treatment, drinking driver, and community samples

	Alcoholism treatment (1) (N = 98)	Drinking drivers (2) (N = 100)	Community sample (3) (N = 82)	F	Significant post hoc comparisons[a]
Any sexual abuse	66	21	35	25.53‡	1,2; 1,3
Exposure	54	13	26	23.50‡	1,2; 1,3
Touch	60	17	21	29.96‡	1,2; 1,3
Penetration	47	7	9	36.45‡	1,2; 1,3
Father					
Verbal aggression	71	43	31	16.76‡	1,2; 1,3
Moderate violence	56	40	35	4.75†	1,3
Severe violence	45	18	13	15.70‡	1,2; 1,3
Mother					
Verbal aggression	67	55	50	3.05*	1,3
Moderate violence	65	49	51	3.10*	NS
Severe violence	46	27	28	4.97†	1,2; 1,3
Parental					
Severe violence and childhood sexual abuse					
Both	45	11	14	21.30‡	1,2; 1,3
Neither	13	57	41	23.56‡	1,2; 1,3

Notes: * $p \leq 0.05$; † $p \leq 0.01$; ‡ ≤ 0.001 [a] based on Tukey's Test

Source: Copyright by Alcohol Research Documentation, Inc., Rutgers Center of Alcohol Studies, Piscataway, NJ.

or family background characteristic that differed between these groups.

Women in treatment with alcohol problems were significantly more likely to report verbal aggression by fathers (67 per cent), compared to women in treatment without alcohol problems (49 per cent) – though neither moderate nor severe violence were significantly different (Miller *et al.* 1993; Miller and Downs 1995). As with childhood sexual abuse, rates of father verbal aggression remained significantly higher for women with alcohol problems even when parental alcoholism was controlled. In another test of the strength of this relationship, when controlling for parental alcohol problems as well as the woman's current level of psychiatric symptomatology, women with alcohol problems were found to have experienced significantly greater father verbal aggression regardless of whether or not they experienced severe partner violence (Downs *et al.* 1992).

Summary

To date, retrospective research among adults strongly suggests that experiences of childhood victimisation are significantly related to the development of alcohol problems in women. Given that father violence, but not mother violence, has been shown to be related to the development of women's alcohol problems, there is a need to control for the gender of the perpetrator in examining these associations. In addition, personal and family background characteristics are important to control when examining these relationships. Further, retrospective research among adults suggests that experiences of childhood victimisation are significantly related to the development of alcohol problems for men as well. Among studies employing retrospective methodologies, stronger and more sophisticated studies have yielded the most consistent support that childhood victimisation is significantly related to the development of alcohol problems for both men and women (Miller and Downs 1995). Conversely, studies of adolescents have shown mixed results between the connections of childhood victimisation and alcohol use. Finally, prospective studies have indicated that childhood victimisation is not related to alcohol problems for men, and only weakly related to alcohol problems for women.

Table 1.8 Percentage experiencing childhood victimisation across treatment groups, with and without alcohol problems, and the community sample

	Treatment, alcohol problems (1) (N = 178)	Treatment, no alcohol problems (2) (N = 92)	Community sample (3) (N = 82)	F	Significant post hoc comparison[a]
Any sexual abuse					
Exposure	70	52	35	15.83‡	1,2; 1,3; 2,3
Touch	58	43	26	12.74‡	1,2; 2,3
Penetration	60	41	21	19.31‡	1,2; 1,3; 2,3
	44	27	9	18.97‡	1,2; 1,3; 2,3
Father					
Verbal aggression	67	49	31	16.54‡	1,2; 1,3; 2,3
Moderate violence	57	46	35	5.88†	1,3
Severe violence	40	27	13	10.59‡	1,3
Mother					
Verbal aggression	73	68	50	7.01†	1,3; 2,3
Moderate violence	71	63	51	4.80†	1,3
Severe violence	49	41	28	5.11†	1,3
Parental					
Severe violence and childhood sexual abuse					
Both	47	37	14	14.24‡	1,3; 2,3
Neither	12	28	41	15.72‡	1,2; 1,3; 2,3

Notes: [a] Based on Tukey's test;† $p \leq 0.01$; ‡ ≤ 0.001

Source: Copyright by Alcohol Research Documentation, Inc., Rutgers Center of Alcohol Studies, Piscataway, NJ.

Substantive and methodological issues

There are several reasons for the contradictory results reported by research on the association between childhood violence and adult alcohol problems. First, research on adolescents and adults may have yielded contradictory results because connections between childhood victimisation and alcohol abuse may not be evident in the adolescent years (Miller and Downs 1995). Sexually or physically abused adolescents may be no more likely to consume alcohol than non-abused adolescents, but are more likely to use drugs or drink at an earlier age, or drink abusively than non-abused adolescents (e.g. Caviola and Schiff 1989; Singer *et al.* 1989). Alcohol problems may require more time to emerge than other sequelae of childhood violence. A diagnosis of alcohol dependence may take several years to develop and thus be more likely to appear in young adulthood rather than adolescence (Miller and Downs 1995). Instead, during adolescence, intervening problems such as post-traumatic stress disorder (PTSD) may develop that ultimately link experiences of childhood violence and alcohol problems.

Second, method variance between prospective and retrospective research may have yielded contradictory results. Prospective research relies on official records for found cases of maltreatment, and cannot be generalised to undiscovered cases – a serious problem since Straus and Gelles (1990) estimated that from 70 per cent to 95 per cent of annual childhood physical abuse cases are unreported. Also, the comparison group in prospective studies is likely to contain a large but unspecified proportion of undiscovered cases of maltreatment. Thus, at best prospective comparison studies conservatively examine differences between abused and non-abused groups. Further, existing prospective work has not yet controlled for gender of the perpetrator, an important omission given that father violence but not mother violence has been consistently found to be related to alcohol problems in our work.

Prospective studies based on found cases include both false negative (failure to report childhood victimisation when it had, in fact, occurred) and false positive (reports of childhood victimisation when none occurred) reports of childhood victimisation (Miller and Downs 1995). Official reports depend on the validity of the data obtained by the investigating worker under conditions of high demand characteristics as well as the validity of that worker's judgments regarding that data. Everson and Boat (1989) found that a subset of social workers were predisposed not to believe children's reports of sexual abuse, a subjective bias resulting in under-reporting of abuse in official records. Retrospective research based on self-report data also includes both false negative and false positive reports (Briere 1992; Williams 1993). Williams (1993, 1994) found that 38 per cent of found cases of childhood sexual abuse later did not report that abuse to researchers using the multiple question and face-to-face interviewing technique recommended by Wyatt and Peters (1986). However, Williams (1993, 1994) found that non-recall was unrelated to past treatment for alcohol abuse or drug abuse.

False positive reports are relatively rare events (Miller and Downs 1995). The most reliable estimates are that from 2 per cent to 8 per cent of childhood sexual abuse reports are false, with the highest rates of false reporting for adolescents (Everson and Boat 1989). An issue more important than false positives is that retrospective research has often consisted of examining those cases that eventually sought treatment. While important to clinicians, this *ex post facto* design cannot be generalised to cases that did not seek treatment.

The strengths of prospective and retrospective studies can be used to complement findings from each methodology. Prospective longitudinal designs can provide data on the course of symptomatology over time as it occurs, without relying on retrospective accounts for the time-ordering of events. Retrospective studies of adults provide the best data available on unreported and untreated cases of childhood sexual abuse and child abuse (Finkelhor 1993). What is needed is a prospective longitudinal examination of unfound cases of maltreatment, but ethical considerations make such a study difficult since once discovered maltreatment cases must be reported – in which case they become found cases. In the absence of such a study, the integration of data from both prospective and retrospective studies is necessary for a full understanding of the links between experiences of childhood violence and the later development of alcohol problems.

Theoretical explanations for the link between childhood violence and adult alcohol problems

The theoretical explanations for the association between experiences of childhood violence and the later development of alcohol-related problems have not been well formulated. One hypothesis is that the development of depression and lower self-esteem during adolescence and adulthood link experiences of childhood violence and later alcohol problems (Downs 1993). Various studies have shown that frequency of corporal punishment (Straus 1993); victimisation from sexual assault (Boney-McCoy and Finkelhor 1993); and sexual abuse (Boisso et al. 1989; Becker et al. 1991) predicted depressive symptoms or lower self-esteem. In a path analysis, Dembo et al. (1989) found that physical and sexual abuse in juvenile delinquents led to drug use via self-derogation.

A second explanation concerns drinking as an escape, which was found to be an important undercurrent in the connection between violent victimisation and the development of alcohol problems in adulthood (Miller et al. 1993). In particular, victims of childhood violence may experience a range of symptoms of post-traumatic stress disorder (Herman 1992) or Type II trauma as outlined by Terr (1991). Boney-McCoy and Finkelhor (1993) found that both sexual abuse and parental violence were related to post-traumatic stress disorder symptoms in both male and females ages 10–16. Also, an inter-relationship between victimisation, alcohol problems, and post-traumatic stress disorder symptomology has been reported (Crime Victims Research and Treatment Center 1992). Alcohol may be used to numb the intense feelings generated by trauma derived from abusive experiences (Gelinas 1983; Herman 1992).

A third explanation reported in the literature, primarily for men, is based on anti-social personality disorder as a link between experiences of childhood violence and the development of alcohol problems in adulthood. Luntz and Widom (1994) reported that childhood parental victimisation experiences were related to a number of lifetime symptoms and diagnosis of anti-social personality disorder, controlling for demographics and arrest history. Anti-social personality disorder has been extensively studied in the US literature on alcohol dependence and found to be one of the more frequent co-occurring diagnoses with alcohol dependence (Hesselbrock et al. 1985; Helzer and Pryzbek 1988; Liskow *et al.* 1991). However, there are serious empirical and definitional problems with this line of theoretical work (see pp. 29–30).

In fact, this link is likely to involve a much broader spectrum of problems than the medical diagnosis of anti-social personality disorder. Aggressive behaviour more generally may be both the sequelae of childhood violence and the precursor of alcohol problems – thus the link between experiences of childhood violence and the development of adulthood alcohol problems. Problems exhibited by adolescent males who have been physically and/or sexually abused include delinquency and sexual acting out (Malamuth *et al.* 1991). Similar problems have been found among boys who observed violence between their parents, for example, behaviour problems (Hughes *et al.* 1989) and aggressive behaviour (Pollock *et al.* 1990).

Finally, conditions within the homes of victimised children must be considered whenever examining the inter-relationships between childhood victimisation and the development of alcohol problems. Parental alcoholism has been found to be a consistent and strong predictor of the development of alcoholism in children (Chassin *et al.* 1991; Babor *et al.* 1992). Given that parental alcohol problems are related to experiences of childhood violence, the combination of multiple negative experiences must be considered in assessing the impact of childhood events on adulthood problems.

IMPLICATIONS OF FINDINGS

The findings of the present study indicate a potential pathway for the inter-generational links between experiences of childhood violence and the development of adulthood alcohol problems for women. First, parental alcohol problems have been found to be related to the perpetration of childhood maltreatment. Also, parental alcohol problems have been found to relate to experiences of childhood sexual abuse for the daughters of parents with alcohol problems. Further, these same experiences of childhood maltreatment have then be found to relate to the development of adulthood alcohol problems for women, placing the next generation of children at risk from experiences of childhood maltreatment, thereby perpetuating the inter-generational cycle of childhood maltreatment and alcohol problems. Other studies have found similar links for men. It is incumbent upon policy-makers and service providers to end this inter-generational cycle.

First, there needs to be sufficient attention and resources provided for the prevention of childhood maltreatment. The children of parents with alcohol problems have an elevated risk of physical abuse from the parent with the alcohol problem and sexual abuse from others outside the nuclear family. Service providers in both the alcoholism and child protection services need to work together to identify these children for early intervention programmes to end the abuse and to provide treatment for its sequelae.

Second, clinicians providing alcoholism and other drug treatment services need to recognise that childhood victimisation is an important experience for most of the women as well as for a majority of the men that they treat. Screening for childhood experiences of physical and sexual abuse needs to be done. Failure to address the importance and meaning of these experiences for those in treatment may contribute to relapse. If men and women have used alcohol as a way of coping with negative feelings generated towards themselves – numbing pain and blurring images of victimisation – or as a way of engaging in aggressive behaviour towards others, removal of the alcohol must be accompanied with support and treatment for these additional issues.

For many treatment programmes, the expertise and experience to provide this type of counselling may not be readily available within the programme. Training of personnel and/or collaborating with family violence and other victimisation service providers may be necessary. Establishing and nurturing an atmosphere in which childhood victimisation experiences can be discussed is important to treatment. For example, standard practices of having women and men together in treatment settings, particularly in group sessions, may not work well for women who have experienced repeated physical and sexual assault from adult males in childhood. Treatment providers need to recognise that each client has the right to control when and to whom she or he reveals her or his personal experiences. Treatment settings that 'schedule' discussion of certain issues in the course of treatment are taking control away from clients. This lack of control occurred during the abusive experience, and if repeated in treatment can make the treatment experience uncomfortably similar to the victimisation experience. Thus, treatment for sexual abuse and other traumatic issues must be voluntary, and under the control of the client.

Third, screening for alcohol and drug problems needs to occur in treatment and intervention settings that provide services for family violence as well as more general victim services. If it is difficult for family violence agencies to address the dual problems of addiction and victimisation, then cooperative structures must be created between these agencies and alcoholism service agencies.

These second and third issues point to the need for inter-organisational structures to encourage coordinated and cooperative models of working together among those engaged in providing services for alcohol problems, family violence, and mental health generally. Not only can this lead to more humane responses, this understanding is key to the development of successful approaches to complex problems in each of these areas. Finally, researchers need to continue to explore the connections between childhood victimisation and alcohol problems. The relationships need to be tested for those at different developmental stages. It would be especially valuable to determine whether the links hold for those from different geographic regions, various cultural backgrounds, more diversified socioeconomic backgrounds, and different nations. Careful testing of the models for how and why childhood victimisation can lead to alcohol problems is needed.

NOTE

DSM-III criteria refer to the criteria for a psychiatric diagnosis of alcohol abuse or dependence based on the Diagnostic and Statistical Manual of Mental Disorders, Third Edition.

REFERENCES

Allen, C. M. and Epperson, D. L. (1993) 'Perpetrator gender and type of child maltreatment: overcoming limited conceptualisations and obtaining representative samples', *Child Welfare*, 72(6): 543–54.
Alterman, A.I. and Cacciola, J. S. (1991) 'The antisocial personality disorder diagnosis in substance abusers: problems and issues', *Journal of Nervous and Mental Disease*, 179(7): 401–9.
American Psychiatric Association Task Force on Nomenclature and Statistics (1980) *Diagnostic and Statistical Manual of Mental Disorders* (3rd edn), Washington, DC: American Psychiatric Association.
Andreasen, N.C. Endicott, J., Spitzer, R.L. and Winokur, G. (1977) 'The

family history method using diagnostic criteria', *Archives of General Psychiatry*, 34: 1229–35.

Babor, T.F., Hofmann, M., DelBoca, F.K., Hesselbrock, V., Meyer, R.E., Dolinsky, Z.S. and Rounsaville, B. (1992) 'Types of Alcoholics, I. Evidence for an empirically derived typology based on indicators of vulnerability and severity', *Archives of General Psychiatry*, 49: 599–608.

Becker, J. V., Kaplan, M. S., Tenke, C. E., and Tartaglini, A. (1991) 'The incidence of depressive symptomatology in juvenile sex offenders with a history of abuse', *Child Abuse and Neglect*, 15: 531–36.

Black, R., and Mayer, J. (1980) 'Parents with special problems: alcoholism and opiate addiction', *Child Abuse and Neglect*, 4: 45–54.

Blane, H. T., Miller, B. A., and Leonard, K. E. (1988) *Intra- and Intergenerational Aspects of Serious Domestic Violence and Alcohol and Drugs*, Washington, DC: National Institute of Justice.

Boisso, C. V., Lutz, D. J., and Gray, S. A. (1989) *Psychological characteristics of adolescent males who have been sexually abused.* Paper presented at the annual meeting of the American Psychological Association, New Orleans, LA, August.

Boney-McCoy, S. and Finkelhor, D. (1993) *The Psychosocial Impact of Violent Victimisation on a National Youth Sample*, Durham, NH: University of New Hampshire.

Briere, J. and Runtz, M. (1987) 'Post sexual abuse trauma: data and implications for clinical practice', *Journal of Interpersonal Violence*, 2: 367–79.

Briere, J., Evans, D., Runtz, M. (1988) 'Symptomatology associated with childhood sexual victimisation in a non-clinical adult sample', *Child Abuse and Neglect*, 12: 51–9.

Briere, J., Evans, D., Runtz, M. and Wall, T. (1988) 'Symptomatology in men who were molested as children: a comparison study', *American Journal of Orthopsychiatry*, 58: 457–61.

Briere, J. (1992) 'Methodological issues in the study of sexual abuse effects', *Journal of Consulting and Clinical Psychology*, 60: 196–203.

Cavaiola, A. A. and Schiff, M. (1989) 'Self-esteem in abused chemically dependent adolescents', *Child Abuse and Neglect*, 13: 327–34.

Chassin, L., Rogosch, F. and Barrera, M. (1991) 'Substance use and symptomatology among adolescent children of alcoholics', *Journal of Abnormal Psychology*, 100: 449–63.

Cloninger, C. R. (1987) 'Neurogenetic adaptive mechanisms in alcoholism', *Science*, 236: 410–16.

Covington, S. S. (1983) 'Sexual experience, dysfunction and abuse: a descriptive study of alcoholic and nonalcoholic women'. PhD dissertation, Cincinnati, Ohio: the Union for Experimenting Colleges and Universities.

Crime Victims Research and Treatment Center (1992) *Rape in America: A Report to the Nation*, Arlington, VA: National Victim Center.

Dembo, R., Dertke, M., Levi, L., Borders, S., Washburn, M. and Schmeidler, J. (1987) 'Physical abuse, sexual victimisation and illicit drug use: a structural analysis among high risk adolescents', *Journal of Adolescence*, 10: 13–33.

Dembo R., Dertke, M., Borders, S., Washburn M. and Schmeidler, J. (1988a) 'The relationship between physical and sexual abuse and tobacco, alcohol, and illicit drug use among youths in a juvenile detention center', *International Journal of the Addictions*, 23(4): 351–78.

Dembo R., Williams, L., Wish, E. D., Dertke, M., Berry, E., Getreu, A., Washburn, M. and Schmeidler, J. (1988b) 'The relationship between physical and sexual abuse and illicit drug use: a replication among a new sample of youths entering a juvenile detention center', *International Journal of the Addictions*, 23(11): 1101–23.

Dembo, R., Williams, L., La Voie, L., Berry, E., Getreu, A., Wish, W.D., Schmeidler, J. and Washburn, M. (1989) 'Physical abuse, sexual victimisation and illicit drug use: replication of a structural analysis among a new sample of high risk youths', *Violence and Victims*, 4: 121–38.

DiLalla, L. F. and Gottesman, I. I. (1991) 'Biological and genetic contributions to violence: Widom's untold tale', *Psychological Bulletin*, 109: 125–29.

Downs, W. R., Miller, B. A. and Gondoli, D. (1987) 'Childhood experiences of parental physical violence for alcoholic women compared with a randomly selected household sample', *Violence and Victims*, 2(4): 81–96.

Downs, W. R., Miller, B. A., Testa, M. and Panek, D. (1992) 'Long-term effects of parent-to-child violence for women', *Journal of Interpersonal Violence*, 7(3): 365–82.

Downs, W. R. (1993) 'Developmental considerations for the effects of childhood sexual abuse', Journal of Interpersonal Violence, 8(3): 331–45.

Downs, W. R. and Miller, B. A. (1994) *Women's Alcohol Problems and Experiences of Partner Violence: A Longitudinal Examination*, Paper presented at the Annual Meeting of the Research Society on Alcoholism, Maui, Hawaii, June.

Everson, M. D. and Boat, B. W. (1989) 'False allegations of sexual abuse by children and adolescents', *Journal of American Academy of Child and Adolescent Psychiatry*, 28(2): 230–35.

Fagan, J. (1993) 'Interactions among drugs, alcohol, and violence', *Violence and the Public's Health*, 12: 65–79.

Famularo, R., Kinscherff, R. and Fenton, T. (1992a) 'Parental substance abuse and the nature of child maltreatment', *Child Abuse and Neglect*, 16: 475–83.

Famularo, R., Kinscherff, R. and Fenton, T. (1992b) 'Psychiatric diagnoses of abusive mothers: a preliminary report', *Journal of Nervous and Mental Disease*, 180(10): 658–61.

Finkelhor, D. (1979) *Sexually Victimized Children*, New York: Free Press.

Finkelkor, D. (1993) 'Answers to important questions about the scope and nature of child sexual abuse'. Unpublished Manuscript, Durham, NH: University of New Hampshire, Family Research Laboratory.

Finkelhor, D. and Baron, L. (1986) 'High-risk children', in D. Finkelhor (ed.), *Sourcebook on Child Sexual Abuse*, Newbury Park, CA: Sage.

Finkelhor, D., Hotaling, G., Lewis, I. A. and Smith, C. (1989) 'Sexual abuse and its relationship to later sexual satisfaction, marital status, religion, and attitudes', *Journal of Interpersonal Violence*, 4: 379–99.

Gelinas, D. (1983) 'The persisting negative effects of incest', *Psychiatry*, 46: 312–32.

Goldston, D. B., Turnquist, D. C. and Knutson, J. F. (1989) 'Presenting problems of sexually abused girls receiving psychiatric services', *Journal of Abnormal Psychology*, 98: 314–17.

Hamberger, L. K. and Hastings, J. E. (1987) *The male batterer and alcohol abuse: differential personality characteristics*. Paper presented at a symposium on The Male Batterer: Alcohol Use, Jealousy, and Consequences of Abuse, Western Psychological Association, Long Beach, CA, April.

Harrison, P. A., Hoffmann, N. G. and Edwall, G. E. (1989a) 'Differential drug use patterns among sexually abused adolescent girls in treatment for chemical dependency', *International Journal of the Addictions*, 24: 499–514.

Harrison, P. A., Hoffmann, N. G. and Edwall, G. E. (1989b) 'Sexual abuse correlates: similarities between male and female adolescents in chemical dependency treatment', *Journal of Adolescent Research*, 4(3): 385–99.

Helzer, J. E. and Pryzbeck, T. R. (1988) 'The co-occurrence of alcoholism with other psychiatric disorders in the general population and its impact on treatment', *Journal of Studies on Alcohol*, 49: 219–24.

Herman, J. L. (1992) *Trauma and Recovery*, New York: Basic Books.

Hesselbrock, V. M., Meyer, R. E. and Keener, R. E. (1985) 'Psychopathology in hospitalized alcoholics', *Archives of General Psychiatry*, 42: 1050–55.

Hill, E. M., Nord, J. L. and Blow, F. C. (1992) 'Young-adult children of alcoholic parents: protective effects of positive family functioning', *British Journal of Addiction*, 87: 1677–90.

Holmes, S. J. and Robins, L. N. (1987) 'The influence of childhood disciplinary experience on the development of alcoholism and depression', *Journal of Child Psychology and Psychiatry and Allied Disciplines*, 28: 399–415.

Holmes, S. J. and Robins, L. N. (1988) 'The role of parental disciplinary practices in the development of depression and alcoholism', *Psychiatry*, 51: 24–36.

Hughes, H. M., Parkinson, D. and Vargo, M. (1989) 'Witnessing spouse abuse and experiencing physical abuse: a "double whammy"?', *Journal of Family Violence*, 4: 197–209.

Ireland, T. and Widom, C. S. (1994) 'Childhood victimisation and risk for alcohol and drug arrests', International Journal of the Addictions, 29(2): 237–74.

Kantor, G. K. (1992) *Violent families and alcohol-abusing families: examining the consequences for children*. Paper presented at the Annual Meeting of the American Society of Criminology, New Orleans, LA, November.

Kantor, G. K. and Straus, M. A. (1990) *Parental drinking and violence and child aggression.* Paper presented at the Annual Meeting of the American Psychological Association, Boston, MA, August.

Kendall-Tackett, K. A., Williams, M. L. and Finkelhor, D. (1993) 'Impact of sexual abuse on children: a review and synthesis of recent empirical studies', *Psychological Bulletin*, 113(1): 164–80.

Kroll, P. D., Stock, D. F. and James, M. E. (1985) 'The behavior of adult alcoholic men abused as children', *Journal of Nervous and Mental Disease*, 173(11): 689–93.

Lanktree, C., Briere, J. and Zaidi, L. (1991) 'Incidence and impact of sexual abuse in a child outpatient sample: the role of direct inquiry', *Child Abuse and Neglect*, 15: 447–53.

Liskow, B., Powell, B. J., Nickel, E. and Penick, E. (1991) 'Antisocial alcoholics: are there clinically significant diagnostic subtypes?', *Journal of Studies on Alcohol*, 52: 62–9.

Luntz, B. K. and Widom, C. S. (1994) 'Antisocial personality disorder in abused and neglected children grown up', *American Journal of Psychiatry*, 151(5): 670–74.

McCord, J. (1983) 'A forty year perspective on effects of child abuse and neglect', *Child Abuse and Neglect*, 7: 265–70.

Malamuth, N. M., Sockloskie, R. J., Koss, M. P. and Tanaka, J. S. (1991) 'Characteristics of aggressors against women: testing a model using a national sample of college students', *Journal of Consulting and Clinical Psychology*, 59: 670–81.

Miller, B. A. (1990) 'The interrelationships between alcohol and drugs and family violence', in M. De La Rosa, E. Y. Lambert, and B. Gropper (eds), *Drugs and Violence: Causes, Correlates, and Consequences*, Monograph 103 (DHHS Pub No. ADM–90–1721), Rockville, MA: National Institute on Drug Abuse.

Miller, B. A. and Downs, W. R. (1993) 'The impact of family violence on the use of alcohol by women', *Alcohol, Health, and Research World*, 17(2): 137–43.

Miller, B. A. and Downs, W. R. (1995) 'Violent victimisation among women with alcohol problems', in M. Galanter (ed.) *Recent Developments in Alcoholism*, Vol. 12, New York: Plenum Press.

Miller, B. A., Downs, W. R., Gondoli, D. and Keil, A. (1987) 'Childhood sexual abuse incidents for alcoholic women versus a random household sample', *Violence and Victims*, 2 (3): 157–92.

Miller, B. A., Downs, W. R. and Testa, M. (1993) 'Interrelationships between victimisation experiences and women's alcohol/drug use', *Journal of Studies on Alcohol*, Supplement No. 11: 109–17.

Orme, T. C. and Rimmer, J. (1981). 'Alcoholism and child abuse: a review, *Journal of Studies on Alcohol*, 42: 273–87.

Pernanen, K. (1981) 'Theoretical aspects of the relationship between alcohol use and crime', in J. J. Collins (ed.) *Drinking and Crime*, New York: Guilford Press.

Peters S. D. (1988) 'Child sexual abuse and later psychological problems', in Wyatt, G. E. and Powell, G. J. (eds), *Lasting Effects of Child Sexual Abuse*, Newbury Park, CA: Sage.

Pollock, V.E., Briere, J., Schneider, L., Knop, J., Mednick, S. A. and Goodwin, D. W. (1990) 'Childhood antecedents of antisocial behaviour: parental alcoholism and physical abusiveness', *American Journal of Psychiatry*, 147: 1290–93.

Radomsky, N. A., (1991) 'The association of parental alcoholism and rigidity with chronic illness and abuse among women', *Journal of Family Practice*, 35: 54–60.

Reider, E., Zucker, R. A., Maguin, E. T., Noll, R. B. and Fitzgerald, H. E. (1989) *Alcohol involvement and violence towards children among high risk families*. Paper presented at the 97th Annual Meeting of the American Psychological Association, New Orleans, August.

Richardson, D. (1981) 'The effect of alcohol on male aggression toward female targets', *Motivation and Emotion*, 5: 333–44.

Robins, L. N., Helzer, J. E., Przybeck, T. R. and Regier, D. A. (1988) 'Alcohol disorders in the community: a report from the Epidemiologic Catchment Area', in R. M. Rose and J. Barrett (eds), *Alcoholism: Origins and Outcome*, New York: Raven.

Rohsenow D. J., Corbett R. and Devine D. (1988) 'Molested as children: a hidden contribution to substance abuse?', *Journal of Substance Abuse Treatment*, 5(1): 13–18.

Schaefer, M. R., Sobieraj, K. and Hollyfield, R. L. (1988) 'Prevalence of childhood physical abuse in adult male veteran alcoholics', *Child Abuse and Neglect*, 12: 141–49.

Schuckit, M. A. (1973) 'Alcoholism and sociopathy: diagnostic confusion', *Journal of Studies on Alcohol*, 34: 157–64.

Sgroi, S. M. (1982) *Handbook of Clinical Intervention in Child Sexual Abuse*, Lexington, MA: Lexington Books.

Singer, M. I., Petchers, M. K. and Hussey D. (1989) 'The relationship between sexual abuse and substance abuse among psychiatrically hospitalized adolescents', *Child Abuse and Neglect*, 13: 319–25.

Steele, C. M. and Josephs, R. A. (1990) 'Alcohol myopia: its prized and dangerous effects', *American Psychologist*, 45: 921–33.

Stein, J. A., Golding, J. M., Siegel, J. M., Burnam, M. A. and Sorenson, S. B. (1988) 'Long-term psychological sequelae of child sexual abuse: the Los Angeles Epidemiologic Catchment Area Study', in Wyatt G. E. and Powell G. J. (eds) *Lasting Effects of Child Sexual Abuse*, Newbury Park, CA: Sage.

Straus, M. A. (1979) 'Measuring intrafamily conflict and violence: the Conflict Tactics Scales (CTS)', *Journal of Marriage and the Family*, 41: 75–86.

Straus, M. A. (1993) 'Corporal punishment of children and depression and suicide in adulthood', in J. McCord (ed.) *Coercion and Punishment in Long Term Perspective*, New York, NY: Cambridge University Press.

Straus M. A. and Gelles, R. J. (1990) 'How violent are American families? Estimates from the National Family Violence Resurvey and other studies', in Straus, M. A. and Gelles R. J. (eds) *Physical Violence in American Families: Risk Factors and Adaptions to Violence in 8,145 Families*, New Brunswick, NJ: Transaction Adaptations.

Straus M. A., Gelles, R. J. and Steinmetz, S. K. (1980) *Behind Closed Doors: Violence in the American Family*, Garden City, NY: Anchor Books.

Swett, C. Jr., Cohen, C., Surrey, J., Compaine, A. and Chavez, R. (1991) 'High rates of alcohol use and history of physical and sexual abuse among women outpatients', *American Journal of Drug and Alcohol Abuse*, 17(1): 49–60.

Terr, L. C. (1991) 'Childhood traumas: an outline and overview', *American Journal of Psychiatry*, 148(1): 10–20.

West, M. O. and Prinz, R. J. (1987) 'Parental alcoholism and childhood psychopathology', *Psychological Bulletin*, 102(2): 204–18.

White, H. R. (1990) 'The drug use–delinquency connection in adolescence', in R. Weisheit (ed.), *Drugs, Crime, and the Criminal Justice System*, Cincinnati, OH: Anderson.

Widom, C. S., Ireland, T. and Glynn, P. J. (1995) 'Alcohol abuse in abused and neglected children followed up: are they at increased risk?' *Journal of Studies on Alcohol*, 56(2): 207–17.

Williams, G. D., Grant, B. F., Harford, T. C. and Noble, J. (1989) 'Epidemiologic Bulletin No. 23: population projections using DSM–III criteria: alcohol abuse and dependence 1990–2000,' *Alcohol Health and Research World*, 13: 366–70.

Williams, L. M. (1993) *Recall of childhood trauma: a prospective study of women's memories of child sexual abuse.* Paper presented at the Annual Meeting of the American Society of Criminology, Phoenix, AZ.

Williams, L. M. (1994) 'Recall of childhood trauma: a prospective study of women's memories of child sexual abuse', *Journal of Consulting and Clinical Psychology*, 62(6): 1167–76.

Williams-Petersen, M. G., Myers, B., Degen, H. M., Knisely, J., Elswick, R. K., Jr. and Schnoll, S. S. (1994) 'Drug-using and non-using women: potential for child abuse, child-rearing attitudes, social support, and affection for expected baby', *International Journal of the Addictions*, 29(12): 1631–43.

Wyatt, G. E. and Peters, S. D. (1986) 'Methodological considerations in research on the prevalence of child sexual abuse', *Child Abuse and Neglect*, 10: 241–51.

Zucker, R. (1986) 'The four alcoholisms: a developmental account of the etiologic process', in Jacob, T., Hill, S. Y. and Baker, T. B. (eds) *Alcohol and Addictive Behavior: Nebraska Symposium on Motivation*, Vol. 34. Lincoln, NE: University of Nebraska Press.

Chapter 2

Alcohol and youth

*Emma Fossey, Wendy Loretto and
Martin Plant*

INTRODUCTION

Alcohol consumption by young people periodically becomes the focus for public concern and mass media attention. During recent years extensive publicity has been accorded to 'lager louts' and to the alleged involvement of heavy drinking in public disorder by young people, especially males (British Medical Association 1986). Such 'moral panics' do not necessarily reflect significant increases in levels of alcohol-related problems amongst the young. Sometimes they even occur at times when youthful drinking habits are stable, or when alcohol consumption may be declining (May 1992). The UK shares with North Western Europe and North America an ambivalence towards alcohol. A commonplace feature of this ambivalence takes the form of trepidation about the real or imagined excesses of younger drinkers. The latter, it is sometimes assumed, are particularly vulnerable in this respect because they are inexperienced and inclined to do silly things.

This chapter sets out to review recent evidence on the nature and scale of alcohol-related problems experienced by young people, set within the wider context of normative patterns of youthful alcohol use. Existing interventions directed at tackling alcohol misuse in this population, consisting predominantly of primary preventative measures relating to policy and education, are also discussed, as are implications for future harm-reduction strategies. For the purposes of this review, attention is concentrated upon individuals aged 21 or younger. Most of the evidence considered relates to the UK, although some more general international evidence is also considered.

LEARNING ABOUT ALCOHOL

Most of the concern surrounding youthful drinking is specifically directed towards those individuals in their late teens and early twenties. As a result, the majority of alcohol education initiatives have been designed for use with young people of secondary school age. However, there is evidence that knowledge and attitudes relating to alcohol and drinking develop at a much earlier stage. In many drinking cultures, children are exposed to alcohol use by their parents, guardians and other significant people in their lives, well before they themselves begin to drink regularly. In Britain over 90 per cent of the adult population consume alcohol to a greater or lesser extent – given this environment it is hardly surprising that children become aware of alcohol from a tender age.

Very little research has focused on the information about alcohol which young children possess and/or their attitudes towards consumption. However, one of the most recent studies conducted in this area (Fossey 1993a; 1993b; 1994) traced the development of alcohol-related cognitions in 238 children aged five-and-a-half to ten-and-a-half years from Scotland and England. This exercise took as its inspiration the classic investigation by Jahoda and Cramond (1972) carried out in Glasgow over twenty years previously. In both cases, a series of game-like activities were designed to elicit young children's perceptions of alcohol.

The children in Fossey's study (1993a) demonstrated a high level of awareness of alcohol. Approximately 95 per cent of all subjects were able to identify beer and/or whisky solely on the basis of smell, with the younger children just as likely as the older ones to be able to do so. A similar proportion were likewise able to recognise and attribute to drunkenness, behaviours commonly associated with intoxication. Indeed, when subjects' expectancies regarding the consequences of drinking were examined, it became apparent that most children equated the consumption of alcohol with drunkenness, irrespective of the actual amount consumed. Again, this tendency was displayed by younger and older subjects alike, in spite of the fact that the latter in particular were aware of a variety of emotional/psychological motives for adult drinking.

This propensity to equate consumption with drunkenness might also help to explain the consistently disapproving attitudes towards adult drinkers displayed by these same subjects (Fossey

1993b). On the whole, the five- to six-year-olds tended to exhibit neutral or slightly negative attitudes towards photographs depicting men and women drinking various alcoholic beverages. However, with rising age, subjects became increasingly critical of drinkers, with the female drinkers eliciting greater disapproval than the male drinkers. Moreover, it was the female subjects who tended to be the more judgemental in this respect. A similar stereotypical bias was apparent in children's perceptions of normative drinking behaviours. While men were generally perceived by subjects to like various alcohol-related activities (drinking beer, drinking wine, drinking whisky, going to the pub), women were perceived only to enjoy drinking wine (Fossey 1994).

In comparison with Jahoda and Cramond's findings, Fossey's results suggest that children are likely to have acquired a greater degree of alcohol knowledge by this young age, than was the case over twenty years previously. This is perhaps of little surprise in view of the marked increases in per capita consumption which have occurred during the intervening years. Nevertheless the pattern of responses – in particular the tendency to discriminate against women drinkers, appears to have remained relatively stable. While this latter trend may seem somewhat at odds with the growing number of women now reporting use of alcohol and the widespread acceptance of the normality of women drinkers, it should be noted that married mothers constitute one of the lowest drinking rate groups (Foster et al. 1990; Plant, M. L. 1990), and as such may form rather less representative female role models in relation to transmitting drinking norms. Such social stereotypes might also be better interpreted in terms of the ways in which children are able to assimilate information, that is, as 'products of normal everyday cognitive processes of social categorisation, social inference and social judgement' (Borgida et al. 1981).

A number of studies conducted predominantly in the US, have attempted to assess whether early childhood perceptions of alcohol can in any way be linked to the drinking habits of the parents. There is some evidence to suggest that children from heavier drinking environments tend to perform more ably on recognition and awareness tasks (Noll and Zucker 1983; Greenberg et al. 1985). These trends are to an extent predictable and do not necessarily give cause for concern. Potentially more worrying however, is evidence from some studies which indicates that children from more extreme drinking environments – that is abstainers or heavy/problem drinking families, may be picking up misguided notions of what constitutes normative drinking behaviour (Jahoda and Cramond 1972; Greenberg *et al.* 1985), or of alcohol expectancies (Miller *et al.* 1990), or may display more extreme attitudes towards drinking (Casswell *et al.* 1985). On the other hand, a number of researchers have failed to establish a direct association between parental drinking habits and children's alcohol-related cognitions. Nor is it clear whether early childhood perceptions can in any way be predictive of future patterns of alcohol use.

LEARNING TO DRINK

The hostility to alcohol that is evident amongst young children is replaced by a widespread enthusiasm for it amongst adolescents and teenagers. An illustration of this transition is presented in a qualitative study conducted by Aitken *et al.* (1988). This examined the perceptions of alcohol advertising held by school pupils at 10, 12, 14 and 16 years old. The authors found that the younger adolescents took a moralistic view of such advertising and disapproved of the products, whereas the same adverts portrayed qualities which were perceived as attractive by the older teenagers. In addition, in their study of 14 to 17 year olds, Davies and Stacey (1972) noted that teenagers typically regarded drinking alcohol as a hallmark of sociability and maturity. In fact non-drinkers were often viewed as unsociable.

A considerable number of studies of youthful drinking habits have been conducted in the UK and Ireland since the late 1970s. Many of these have recently been reviewed by several authors (May 1992; Plant and Plant 1992; Lister Sharp 1994). Although some findings have been provided by observational studies (e.g. Dorn 1983; Dean 1990), most information on this topic has been collected by the use of large-scale surveys based on self-reports.

Surveys are inevitably flawed by refusal to cooperate, by non-contact with some of the potential respondents, and by inaccurate reporting by those who do cooperate. Such inaccuracy may be due to poor recall, to deliberate deception or to a combination of both. It has been concluded that such survey data are frequently distorted by under-reporting (Pernanen 1974; Midanik 1982; Plant *et al.* 1985). In addition, as emphasised by Marsh *et al.* (1986), there is evidence that some adolescents, particularly young boys, may exaggerate their alleged alcohol consumption levels.

Nevertheless these studies provide a useful and fairly consistent picture. They indicate that most teenagers in the UK do consume alcoholic beverages. Several studies have shown that around one-third of boys and girls are drinking regularly by the ages of 14 to 15 years old, and that very few British teenagers have not consumed alcohol by the age of 16 (Plant et al. 1985; Marsh et al. 1986; Plant et al. 1990; Plant and Foster 1991; Loretto 1994a, 1994b). In her review of the literature, Lister Sharp (1994) concluded that by the age of 16 years old, 90 per cent of young people in Great Britain will have tasted alcoholic drinks.

The precise proportion of abstainers fluctuates between studies, perhaps due in part to the difficulties associated with data collection as noted above. For example, a national study of 14 to 16 year olds in English state schools revealed that only 4 per cent of a sample of 7009 teenagers had never tasted alcohol (Plant et al. 1990). A parallel study of Scottish teenagers indicated that only 3 per cent had never done so (Plant and Foster 1991). However, what all these studies do show is that drinking is normal behaviour amongst adolescents and teenagers.

A considerable amount of information about adolescent drinking habits has been provided by a survey of 13 to 17 year olds in England, Wales and Scotland (Marsh et al. 1986). In reporting the results of this study, the authors highlighted some differences in behaviour between the countries. They found that in England and Wales, the majority of adolescents had consumed their first 'proper' alcoholic drink (i.e. not just a sip) by the age of 13. Some 18 per cent of 13-year-old boys and 25 per cent of 13-year-old girls had never tasted alcohol or had never consumed an alcoholic drink. It was noted that Scottish adolescents commenced their drinking careers later than their English and Welsh peers but subsequently caught up with them. At 13 years of age, 29 per cent of Scottish males and 43 per cent of Scottish females had never had a whole alcoholic drink. However, by the age of 17, only 7 per cent of girls and 9 per cent of boys in all three countries purported to abstain from alcohol.

National differences have also been reported by Marsh et al., in relation to quantity of alcohol typically consumed. These authors noted:

In Scotland the pattern is again quite different. Not only are young Scots slower to take up drinking but, having done so, they drink less often than do their peers in England and Wales.

(1986: 11)

However, the main regional differences within the UK occur when the drinking patterns of England, Wales and Scotland are compared to those in Northern Ireland. In her review, Lister Sharp noted:

The situation in Northern Ireland is somewhat different [from that in mainland Britain]. In a survey of secondary school pupils two thirds of the boys and over three quarters of the girls reported not drinking at all or only very occasionally.

(1994:1)

Two surveys were undertaken for the Department of Health and Social Services, Northern Ireland in 1988 and 1990 (Craig 1989; Craig *et al.* 1991). When the results of these studies were compared to surveys carried out on the mainland (e.g. Marsh *et al.* 1986), it was found that Northern Irish young people are less likely to have tasted alcohol or to be current drinkers. The first of these Northern Irish studies surveyed school pupils aged between 11 and 17 and reported overall abstinence rates of 39 per cent for males and 60 per cent for females; the second included only those in the 11 to 15-year-old range, of whom half of the males and nearly two-thirds of the females had never consumed a whole alcoholic drink. The differences between the figures produced from these reports are probably due to the different age groups surveyed. Both reported similar drinking prevalence levels for those respondents aged 11. They indicated that 80 per cent of males and 90 per cent of females aged 11 had not consumed alcohol. The 1989 study further showed that the proportion of drinkers among the 17-year-old age group had increased to 82 per cent of the boys and 66 per cent of the girls. The second (1991) study reported 78 per cent and 62 per cent for its 15 year old males and females respectively.

A recent survey of 11 to 12 year olds and 15 to 16 year olds in Scotland and Northern Ireland supported these differences (Loretto 1994a). It was shown that, overall 20 per cent (18 per cent of males; 23 per cent of females) of the Scottish respondents had never consumed a whole drink of alcohol; the corresponding figure for the Northern Irish study group was 25 per cent (19 per cent of males; 38 per cent of females).

Thus, although available evidence indicates that very few teenagers in England, Wales and Scotland do not drink alcohol, a higher proportion of those in Northern Ireland are non-drinkers, consistent with the 'drier' and more polarised drinking cultures of that country. In this respect, Ireland is similar to the US where a substantial minority of adults are abstainers.

In terms of quantities of alcohol consumed, it has been demonstrated that the majority of young drinkers do consume relatively modest amounts. While boys have generally been shown to drink greater amounts than girls of the same age, most studies of youthful alcohol consumption have demonstrated that a substantial minority of teenagers of both sexes report drinking relatively heavily. For example in their surveys of English and Scottish 14 to 16 year olds, Plant and colleagues found that the former survey indicated that 9.7 per cent of boys and 5.1 per cent of girls claimed to have imbibed 11 or more units on their last drinking occasion. The corresponding proportions of Scottish teenagers were 18.9 per cent and 10.3 per cent – supporting the conclusion that Scottish teenagers were more likely than their English counterparts to drink heavily. However, once again the most marked differences occur between those countries that make up the UK mainland and Northern Ireland. When the results of the 1989 DHSS study were compared to that conducted in mainland Britain by Marsh *et al.* (1986) it was found that during the week preceding the surveys, 60 per cent of Northern Irish males and 32 per cent of females from the Province had consumed more than 10 units of alcohol. These figures compare to 38 per cent of males and 13 per cent of females in England and Wales, and to 40 per cent of males and 22 per cent of females in Scotland. From these studies it can be concluded that Scottish teenagers were more likely than those south of the border to drink relatively large amounts and those from Northern Ireland drink even greater quantities than the Scots.

Similar national differences were also highlighted in Loretto's comparative study of Northern Irish and Scottish young people (1994a, 1994b). Using the procedures adopted by Plant and Foster (1991) and Plant *et al.* (1990), details of the most recent occasion's alcohol consumption were used to classify respondents as 'light' and 'heavy' drinkers. Male 'heavy drinkers' were defined as those who had consumed 11 or more units on their last drinking occasion; females eight or more units. It was found that the Northern Irish study group contained a significantly higher proportion of 'heavy drinkers' This was true for both males and females. In Scotland 9 per cent of boys were classed as 'heavy' drinkers – this figure was doubled for Northern Irish males. The differences between the girls in each of the countries were not as marked (Scotland 11 per cent; Northern Ireland 16 per cent) but were still proved to be statistically significant, that is, they were unlikely to have happened by chance.

As noted above, the proportion of teenage drinkers increases with age. It has also been shown that the amount of alcohol consumed increases with age. In Loretto's study, only 3 per cent of males and 1 per cent of females aged 11 to 12 were classed as 'heavy' drinkers. The corresponding figures for the 14- to 16-year-old age group were 26 per cent and 27 per cent. From the studies conducted by Plant and colleagues, it is evident that the proportion of 'heavy' drinkers also increases markedly between the ages of 14 and 16. Amongst males in England the proportion who had reportedly consumed 11 or more units on their last drinking occasion rose from 5.4 per cent to 13.5 per cent. Amongst females the proportion who had consumed eight or more units rose from 7.1 per cent to 15 per cent. However, it is at this stage that effects of gender on increases in consumption tend to diverge. For example, in a four-year follow-up survey of 15 and 16 year olds, Plant *et al.* (1985), found that whereas consumption by males continued to rise during this four-year period, consumption by females remained stable. This could imply that females are more mature in this respect as they attain adult consumption patterns at an earlier age.

A further correlate of 'heavy' teenage drinking which has received some attention is that of family background. A study of 15 to 16 year olds in the Lothian region showed that individuals who had been raised by single parents were heavier drinkers than those who had been raised by two parents or guardians (Plant *et al.* 1985). The heaviest drinkers were teenage boys who had been raised by lone fathers.

In their meta-analysis, mainly of studies conducted in the US, Foxcroft and Lowe (1991) emphasised the importance of parental support and control in the formation of 'safe' adolescent drinking practices. In their own study of adolescent drinkers (Lowe and Foxcroft 1993) the authors further noted:

> Although most young people drink within the normal range, those with alcohol-deviant behaviours (non-drinkers and heavy drinkers) seem more likely to emerge from families where home environment and dynamics are more extreme.
>
> (1993: 205)

Evidence from reviews undertaken by May (1992) and Lister Sharp (1994) shows that, in general, as teenagers grow older, they move from drinking in their own homes to drinking with friends in other places. In this vein, a range of studies (e.g. Davies and Stacey 1972; Marsh et al. 1986; Ghodsian and Power 1987; Craig 1989; Loretto 1994b, 1994c) have examined variables relating to drinking venue, drinking companions and preferred leisure activities, and how these affect styles of drinking.

In brief, the conclusion reached from the findings is that drinking outside the home and in the company of peers, rather than parents, is related to higher alcohol consumption. Moreover, the national differences in levels of alcohol consumption are also reflected in the choice of drinking location and companions. For example, data from the study undertaken by Marsh et al. show that such age-related changes took place at an earlier age amongst the Scottish drinkers. Moreover, the results from the DHSS study in Northern Ireland demonstrated that the proportions drinking in unspecified places (e.g. in parks, wasteland and in streets) were much higher there at each age from 13 to 15 years old than in Scotland, England or Wales. The young people from Northern Ireland were less likely to consume alcohol in the company of parents or other relatives, and more likely to prefer the company of peers. Furthermore, at every age, and for both genders, young people in Northern Ireland were more likely than their mainland British counterparts to be solitary drinkers. Loretto's data (1994a, 1994b) supported these differences between the countries.

With regard to lifestyle variables, in their survey of teenagers and alcohol use, Davies and Stacey (1972) suggested that young people are less likely to smoke and drink if they play a sport and attend youth clubs than if they regularly go to parties and dances. However, the effects of participation in different types of leisure activities on levels of alcohol consumption do not seem to be clear cut. The findings of Davies and Stacey were supported only for females in Loretto's (1994c) study. In their four-area study (Kirkcaldy, Liverpool, Sheffield and Swindon), Roberts and Parsell (1990) found no significant relationships between levels of alcohol consumption and levels of participation in 'dry' leisure activities. Individuals who played sports, went to cinemas, etc. were neither more nor less likely to be frequent drinkers than those with little involvement in such activities.

In the Loretto study it was demonstrated that heavier drinkers were most likely to frequently take part in alcohol-related activities. These included attending parties and discos, visiting pubs and also drinking in other contexts. Not surprisingly, the popularity of such pastimes increased with age. In their survey of 15 to 16 year olds, Coffield et al. (1986) found that licensed premises were among that age group's favourite meeting places.

Finally in this section, the national studies of English and Scottish 14 to 16 year olds (Plant et al. 1990; Plant and Foster 1991) included an examination of teenagers who were relatively 'heavy' drinkers. The latter were distinctive in a number of ways. Heavier drinkers were significantly more likely than other teenagers to have last consumed alcohol with a mixed group of friends. In contrast, lighter drinkers were more likely to have drunk in the company of their parents. Female heavy drinkers were more likely than other females to endorse the view that alcohol increases alertness, that drinking is good for you, that it helps you to talk to the opposite sex, to mix more easily with others, and other positive statements. They were also more likely to agree that they sometimes drank because they were bored. Male heavy drinkers were also more likely than other males to agree with such statements (Plant et al. 1990).

Thus, overall survey evidence indicates that the majority of teenagers in the UK do consume alcohol, but in moderation. Several researchers (e.g. Plant and Foster 1991; May 1992) have even commented on the normality of alcohol consumption among the young, and have emphasised that drinking habits amongst British teenagers have remained relatively stable during the last ten years. The drinking habits of this age group are part of a more general socialisation and coming of age in a society in which drinking is considered to be an important facet of mature and sociable behaviour, and it must be stressed that the great majority learn to drink without serious mishap. Nevertheless, there is reason to be concerned about the drinking habits of a minority of young people.

ALCOHOL-RELATED PROBLEMS

Intoxication and related consequences

As stated above, most of those young people who drink generally consume light to moderate quantities and do not experience serious adverse consequences. Indeed, a growing body of international evidence indicates that light to intermediate levels of alcohol consumption have a protective effect upon rates of premature mortality (e.g. Gronbaek *et al.* 1994; Plant 1994a). In spite of this, some of those who drink do so in ways that lead to adverse consequences, either to themselves or to others. Most of this harm is attributable to acute or periodic heavy or inappropriate drinking or to intoxication rather than to chronic heavy alcohol intake.

Surveys consistently show that a high proportion of adolescent and teenage drinkers sometimes drink to intoxication and experience 'low level' adverse effects such as hangovers, headaches and nausea. The survey by Marsh *et al.* (1986) indicated that youthful intoxication was commonplace. Amongst 13 year olds in England and Wales who were drinkers, 39 per cent of boys and 40 per cent of girls reported having been drunk once; 24 per cent of boys and 14 per cent of girls had been drunk more than once. Amongst 17 year olds, the proportions of those who had experienced intoxication more than once rose to 53 per cent of boys and 30 per cent of girls. In Scotland intoxication was reported by similar proportions. Once again comparisons with Northern Ireland revealed that drinkers there were more likely than their peers in England, Scotland and Wales to have consumed alcohol to intoxication. Two-thirds of Northern Irish drinkers admitted to having been 'slightly' drunk, and almost 40 per cent to having been 'very' drunk. Thus it is clear that intoxication is strongly associated with youthful drinking and is also often considered as 'normal' behaviour amongst teenagers. Dean (1990) has reported that drinking to intoxication is considered as desirable behaviour amongst young people in the Western Isles of Scotland.

An example of the types of adverse consequences associated with youthful drinking has been described by Plant *et al.* (1985).

These authors reported that, amongst 15- to 16-year-old drinkers, 31 per cent of males and 26 per cent of females had experienced hangovers. Some teenagers had also experienced more serious consequences. In this study, 2 per cent of males and 1 per cent of females reported being advised by their doctors to drink less; 6 per cent of males and 3.5 per cent of females stated that they had been worried about their own drinking. Approximately one-fifth of those surveyed reported having had disagreements with their parents that they attributed to their own drinking, 3 per cent of males and 2 per cent of females reported having missed a day's school due to drinking.

The survey by Marsh *et al.* (1986) reinforces the conclusion that many teenage drinkers experience at least minor adverse consequences from their drinking. For example, amongst those aged 13 in Scotland, 28 per cent of boys and 16 per cent of girls reported having been sick due to drinking. These proportions rose to 47 per cent and 28 per cent respectively amongst those aged 17 years. Amongst various sub-groups of Scottish teenagers a minority reported feeling so ill after drinking that they had not gone into work or school (the proportions ranged from 4 per cent of 13-year-old girls to 20 per cent of 17-year-old boys).

These authors also noted that youthful intoxication is frequently associated with 'anti-social' behaviour. Their evidence indicated that up to a quarter of those they surveyed had been in fights, arguments, had upset their parents or had recalled feeling that they should not have gone home. Approximately 10 per cent of boys reported having been involved in vandalism or been noticed by the police due to drinking too much.

However, many of those who, at some time in their lives, experience such adverse consequences are not habitually heavy drinkers. Two important general points should be highlighted. The first is that alcohol-related problems are by no means the sole preserve of the young. It should be emphasised that most teenage 'heavy drinking' involves periodic drinking to intoxication. Popular tabloid newspaper and other popular mass media reports have sometimes referred to 'teenage alcoholism'. In fact chronic heavy drinking, alcohol dependence or 'alcoholism' are rare amongst people below the age of 21. Most of those who seek help from services for problem drinking or 'alcoholism' are above the age of 21 and the majority are in the age range 30 to 60. Second, levels of alcohol-related problems commonly fluctuate in line with changes in general levels of per capita alcohol consumption. Both the UK and Ireland are medium consumption level countries. Many factors influence per capita alcohol consumption. These factors include fashion, tradition, religion, culture, price, availability and disposable income.

Underage drinking in licensed premises

A further alcohol-related problem associated exclusively with young people is that of underage drinking in licensed premises. In the UK it is legal for people aged five and above to consume alcohol, provided that they do not do so in licensed premises. The legal age of alcohol purchase and consumption in the latter is 18. Young people may enter bars, subject to the licensee's permission, once they are 14 years of age in England, Scotland and Wales. The corresponding age in Northern Ireland is 18. People aged 16 to 18 may buy beer, perry and cider (and wine in Scotland) to consume with a meal in a dining room or separate eating area in licensed premises (Lister Sharp 1994). It is clear that a substantial proportion of young people frequent licensed establishments, and buy and consume alcohol there. Survey findings show that between 10 and 20 per cent of 13 year olds report that their usual location for drinking is in a public bar, club or disco. The proportion drinking in these establishments rises steadily with age, until at 17 years of age, between 50 and 90 per cent of young people choose licensed places in which to conduct their drinking (Marsh et al. 1986).

The extent of under-age drinking in licensed premises has been reviewed by Lister Sharp (1994). She noted that this phenomenon is more prevalent in England than in Scotland, Wales or Northern Ireland. Some gender differences were also observed: 'Within countries, boys and girls appear equally likely to drink in pubs in England and Wales or Northern Ireland; however, Scottish boys seem to do so more than girls' (1994: 5).

Lister Sharp further noted that far more young people are found guilty of being drunk than are convicted of consuming alcohol illegally on licensed premises. She observed that the number of Scottish convictions for selling alcohol to minors remained fairly stable during recent years. Nevertheless, the number of people under 18 who were convicted for underage alcohol purchase fell from 1,242 in 1973 to only 44 in 1991. In England and Wales fewer than 2,000 people have been convicted annually of underage alcohol purchase in recent years. In addition, fewer than 500 have been convicted annually of selling alcohol to minors since 1981. Up to 5,000 individuals under the age of 18 have been annually convicted or cautioned in relation to drunkenness offences in England and Wales. Such offences reached a peak in 1983. In Scotland there has been a steady decline since 1974 in the numbers of young people convicted of under-age purchase. Other youthful alcohol offences in Scotland have also declined or have remained rare and stable. No recent comparable data are available for Northern Ireland. These figures led Lister Sharp to conclude that: 'overall, the conviction rates are grossly out of step with the general consistently high level of underage drinking reported by young people themselves' (1994: 6).

Although there is some suggestion that premature initiation into pub culture can lead to heavier drinking later on in life (Ghodsian and Power 1987), this relationship is by no means clear cut (Bagnall 1991a; Plant et al. 1985). Moreover, there is some concern that a substantial purge on under-age drinking could have a displacement effect. If the young people could no longer drink in bars they would simply move to other locations such as parks and street corners (Tuck 1989). Supporters of the displacement theory argue that it is surely better to have teenagers drinking in an environment where there is some regulation – as is the cases in bars – than to force them to drink in completely unregulated contexts.

Morbidity and mortality

The heavy, inappropriate consumption of alcohol is associated with a variety of acute and chronic health problems. These have been reviewed in detail elsewhere (e.g. Collins 1982; Royal College of Psychiatrists 1986; Giesbrecht et al. 1989). With regard to young people, levels of alcohol-related deaths associated with chronic disease appear to be very low. Plant and Plant (1992), reviewing levels of alcohol problems amongst British youth, reported that the annual number of such deaths is tiny. For example, in 1988 three males and five females aged 24 or younger died of chronic liver disease in England and Wales. This condition is often alcohol-related. In addition, a small number of young people die annually from accidental alcohol poisoning.

Of greater concern for this age group is the high incidence of accidental injuries and deaths among young people, which occur as a result of acute intoxication. The Royal College of Psychiatrists (1986) and Giesbrecht *et al.* (1989) have cited evidence indicating that a high proportion of accidental injuries involve people who had been drinking, and that many were intoxicated when they were hurt. Moreover, drinking continues to be involved with a substantial proportion of road traffic accidents. Approximately 1000 people aged 19 or under die each year in road traffic accidents in Britain. Available evidence suggests that many of these deaths are alcohol-related.

On a more optimistic note, the period between 1979 and 1989 saw a substantial fall in the involvement of alcohol in vehicle driver fatalities in Britain. This decrease was especially pronounced amongst younger drivers. For example the proportion of two-wheeled vehicle drivers aged 16 to 19 killed in accidents who were above the legal blood alcohol level fell from 26 per cent to 13 per cent. Amongst drivers of cars and other vehicles the corresponding rate fell from 34 per cent to 11 per cent (Department of Transport 1990). However, it should be noted that this pleasing trend has been accompanied by an increase in alcohol-related deaths amongst pedestrians (Christie 1994).

Alcohol-related crime

Many offenders and victims of crime are subsequently found to have been consuming alcohol prior to the criminal activity. However, as reviewed by Collins (1982), the connection between drinking and crime is frequently unclear, and the precise role of alcohol, if any, is often a matter for conjecture. The picture is often complicated by the fact that both heavier drinkers and known offenders are typically young men from the same age group, that is 16 to 24 years.

In spite of this, crimes of violence do sometimes appear to be partly attributable to drinking. Evidence from Sweden (Lenke 1990) has indicated that rates of homicides tend to change in accordance with fluctuations in alcohol consumption in Swedish society. Similarly temporary disruptions to the availability of alcohol, for example through strike action, appear to produce reductions in a variety of violent criminal acts (Room 1983; Osterberg and Sirrka-Liisa 1991). What is less clear is whether such trends are due to a real reduction in alcohol-related aggression or rather to a fall in the number of potential intoxicated victims.

Alcohol and risk-taking

An extensive body of evidence supports the conclusion that young people who drink heavily are also particularly likely to engage in a variety of other potentially risky behaviours. The latter include tobacco smoking, illicit drug use, and unprotected sex. The American sociologist, Goode, has noted:

> people who use illegal drugs, marijuana [cannabis] especially, are fundamentally the same people who use alcohol and cigarettes – they are a little further along the same continuum. People who abstain from liquor and cigarettes are far less likely to use marijuana than people who smoke and or drink.
>
> (1972)

Although the first part of this statement is highly contentious – as yet there is no conclusive proof that drinking alcohol or smoking tobacco will progress to experimentation with other (illicit) drugs – the latter half is supported by evidence from surveys. For example, in her survey of young people in Scotland and Northern Ireland, Loretto (1994b) demonstrated that being a drinker increased the odds of smoking by a factor of eight, and the odds of ever having tried illicit drugs four and a half times.

The advent of the HIV/AIDS pandemic has aroused concern about the possible connection between drinking and high-risk sexual behaviour. Several investigations have examined the alcohol–sex connection amongst a variety of different study groups of adolescents, teenagers and other young adults, including those working as prostitutes (e.g. Robertson and Plant 1986; Morgan Thomas 1990). This evidence has recently been reviewed (Plant 1994b; World Health Organisation 1994). It is concluded that most studies of young heterosexuals indicate that people who are heavy drinkers are especially likely to engage in high-risk or unprotected sex. In spite of this, it has not been demonstrated that an individual's sexual behaviour on specific occasions is influenced by drinking prior to sexual contact: all that can be concluded is that some people are by nature more generally inclined to take risks.

Nevertheless, this contrasts with the fact that many young drinkers report that they are less sexually inhibited and more likely to take risks after they have consumed alcohol. Studies amongst gay men have produced inconsistent results, although some also suggest that heavier drinkers are in general inclined to take more sexual risks than are other people. It should, however, be emphasised that available evidence does not support the popular view (or misconception) that drinking *per se* promotes unsafe sex.

Young people who drink heavily are also likely to engage in other potentially high-risk activities. These include driving without seat-belts and dangerous sports (Plant and Plant 1992). It is important to note however that the connection between drinking and other activities is frequently attributable to the fact that drinking is a facet of social activity. Moreover, alcohol consumption is very often purely a secondary component of such social activity, rather than its primary focus.

DOES YOUTHFUL HEAVY DRINKING LEAD TO LATER PROBLEMS?

One concern about heavy drinking amongst adolescents or other young people is that it might lead to the development of chronic heavy drinking or alcohol-related problems later in life. Two British studies have followed groups of young people for periods of seven years (Ghodsian and Power 1987) and ten years (Plant *et al.* 1985; Bagnall 1991a). These studies revealed that there were only low levels of association between teenage drinking habits and later patterns of alcohol use. Nevertheless, Ghodsian and Power did interpret their results as supporting the view that teenagers who drink heavily are particularly likely to be heavy drinkers later in life. Plant, Bagnall and their co-authors (1991) did not reach this conclusion from their study. However they did suggest that teenage heavy drinkers were more likely than others to use a wider range of illicit drugs later in life.

A review by Fillmore (1988) has examined the international evidence from prospective studies of individual's drinking habits over time. She concluded that there is generally little continuity and that drinking careers change considerably with increasing age. Reviews of survey evidence (e.g. Plant and Plant 1992; May 1992, 1993c) have noted that consumption of alcohol by young males peaks between the ages of 19 and 21; the corresponding age for females is lower, at 18 years old. Thereafter, drinking patterns appear to 'mature out'. This process involves decreases both in amounts of alcohol consumed and in drinking frequency, and is particularly noticeable amongst males who tend to experience higher peak levels of consumption.

PREVENTION AND CONTROL

Much thought and discussion has been devoted to the problem of how to prevent or curb levels of problematic drinking amongst young people. The ideal solution, perhaps, would be to employ health education in order to warn the young of the potential dangers of intoxication and inappropriate drinking and thereby to discourage such behaviour. In fact many such initiatives have been implemented and directed at the young, especially adolescents and teenagers. Most of these initiatives have never been assessed, while those which have do not provide encouraging results. Review evidence tends to confirm the general failure of health education to influence youthful drinking habits, at least in the short term (Kalb 1975; Kinder *et al.* 1980; Schaps *et al.* 1981; Bandy and President 1983; Coggans *et al.* 1989; Bagnall 1991b; May 1993b; Plant, M. L. 1994). Some initiatives have even been found to be counter-productive, though it should be stressed that the latter refers to an increase in drinking, and not necessarily to a rise in problem drinking.

The results of studies of younger children highlight two important points in this respect. The first is that children are learning about alcohol from a very early age. Most formal alcohol education initiatives have tended to ignore this age group, preferring instead to concentrate on adolescents. The usefulness of directing prevention messages at a group of individuals for whom drinking is already becoming a regular, and frequently non-problematic, activity, is questionable. However, targetting young children before their own involvement with alcohol reaches significant levels might be a more effective strategy.

Second, it is evident that parents play a crucial role in shaping children's initial ideas about alcohol. Indeed, in a recent survey of 736 parents in three areas of Britain (Fossey and Miller 1994), the majority of respondents felt that parents had the primary responsibility of educating their young children about alcohol, while the school was seen as playing a secondary, though equally necessary, role. The messages which children receive from parents may conflict or concur with the messages provided by formal alcohol education. Surely then, a more constructive option for primary intervention would be to enlist the cooperation of parents.

In relation to educational messages, one further point should be introduced. Many of the surveys of teenage drinking have shown that differences in drinking patterns exist between the countries of the UK. In particular, the information relating to Northern Ireland suggests that the culture of this country is much more ambivalent towards the use of alcohol than are the cultures of England, Scotland or Wales (Craig 1989; Craig et al. 1991; Loretto 1994a, 1994b). Such ambivalence, as noted by Bales (1962) may serve to foster both the avoidance and the heavy problematic use of alcohol amongst both adolescents and older drinkers. It is thus argued that in order for alcohol education initiatives to be effective, they must be tailored to the culture in which they are being implemented.

More encouragingly, recent experience with drinking and driving suggests that if public opinion is informed and aroused, dramatic changes are possible. There has clearly been a great hardening of public attitudes towards driving while intoxicated, as well as an impressive behavioural change. The reasons for the marked fall in driver deaths, especially amongst those involving young people, are unclear. However, it may be that while education does have an important role to play, reinforcement by means of concomitant changes in control policy are also necessary. For as May (1993c) has observed, such offences have been viewed increasingly seriously by police, courts and insurance companies.

Similarly, local action to enforce liquor licensing laws or to enforce local bylaws have also sometimes led to a substantial fall in levels of public disorder and offences by young people (Jeffs and Saunders 1983; Ilgunas 1993). It is interesting to note that under-age drinking on licensed premises occurs widely.

Adolescent drinking is both normal and legal – the latter provided it does not occur on licensed premises. Furthermore, for many, their use of alcohol remains unproblematic. In this context, education and policy initiatives can be seen to be directed at the small minority of young people whose drinking is seen to be problematic. However, it is this group of individuals who will be particularly resistant to either type of preventive strategy.

As several commentators have noted, controls, such as local bylaws, often appear to do little more than shift the problem to another location (Davies and Stacey 1972; Ilgunas 1993). It is for these and other reasons that May (1993c) has highlighted the crucial role of the primary health care team, both in terms of identification of and intervention for, those individuals whose problematic drinking styles may place them at risk.

This chapter has outlined the patterns of youthful drinking behaviour in the UK. It has been stressed that most young drinkers are able to consume alcohol without incurring any undesirable effects. Moreover, review evidence indicates that such behaviours have changed little over the past twenty years. However, these data also suggest that a small proportion of adolescents and teenagers do consume alcohol to levels which are cause for concern. The success and effectiveness of a variety of preventative and control measures in relation to adolescent drinking have been discussed, and some ways forward have been suggested.

REFERENCES

Aitken, P., Leather, D. S. and Scott, A. C. (1988) *Ten to Fourteen Year Olds and Alcohol: A Developmental Study in the Central Region of Scotland*, Edinburgh: HMSO.

Bagnall, G. (1991a) 'Alcohol and drug use in a Scottish cohort: ten years on', *British Journal of Addiction*, 86: 895–904.

Bagnall, G. (1991b) *Educating Young Drinkers*, London: Tavistock/ Routledge.

Bales, R. F. (1962) 'Attitudes toward drinking in the Irish culture', in D. J. Pittman and C. R. Snyder (eds) *Society, Culture and Drinking Patterns*, London: John Wiley.

Bandy, P. and President, P. A. (1983) 'Recent literature on drug and prevention and mass media', *Journal of Drug Education*, 13: 255–71.

Borgida, E., Locksley, A. and Brekke, N. (1981) 'Social stereotypes and social judgement', in N. Cantor and J. F. Kihlstrom (eds) *Personality, Cognition and Social Interaction*, Hillsdale, NJ: Erlbaum.

British Medical Association (1986) *Young People and Alcohol*, London: British Medical Association.

Cameron, D. and Plant, M. A. (eds) (1994) *Alcohol and Young People: Learning to Cope*, London: Portman Group.

Casswell, S., Brasch, P., Gilmore, L. and Silva, P. (1985) 'Children's attitudes to alcohol and awareness of alcohol-related problems', *British Journal of Addiction*, 83: 223–7.

Christie, M. (1994) Personal Communication.

Coffield, F., Borrill, C. and Marshall, S. (1986) *Growing Up at the Margins*,

Milton Keynes: Open University Press.

Coggans, N., Shewan, D., Henderson, M., Davies, J. B. and O'Hagan, F. (1989) *National Evaluation of Drug Education in Scotland*, Centre for Occupational and Health Psychology, University of Strathclyde.

Collins, J. J. Jnr. (ed.) (1982) *Drinking and Crime*, London: Tavistock.

Craig, J. for Department of Health and Social Services, (1989) *Drinking Amongst Schoolchildren in Northern Ireland: A Survey Report*, Belfast: HMSO.

Craig, J., Francis, D. and McWhirter, L. for Department of Health and Social Services (1991) *Smoking and Drinking amongst 11–15 year olds in Northern Ireland in 1990*, Belfast: HMSO.

Davies, J. B. and Stacey, B. (1972) *Teenagers and Alcohol*, London: HMSO.

Dean, A. (1990) 'Culture and community: Drink and soft drugs in Hebridean youth culture', *Sociological Review*, 38: 517–65.

Department of Transport (1990) *Blood Alcohol Levels in Fatalities in Great Britain 1988*, Transport and Road Research Laboratory.

Dorn, N. (1981) 'Social analysis of education and the media', in G. Edwards and C. Busch (eds) *Drug Problems in Britain: A Review of Ten Years*, London: Academic Press.

Dorn, N. (1983) *Alcohol, Youth and the State: Drinking Practices, Controls and Health Education*, London: Croom Helm.

Edwards, G. and Busch, C. (eds) (1981) *Drug Problems in Britain: A Review of Ten Years*, London: Academic Press.

Fillmore, K. M. (1988) *Alcohol Across The Life Course*, Toronto: Addiction Research Foundation.

Fossey, E. (1993a) 'Young children and alcohol: a theory of attitude development', *Alcohol and Alcoholism*, 28: 485–98.

Fossey, E. (1993b) 'Identification of alcohol by smell amongst young children: an objective measure of early learning in the home', *Drug and Alcohol Dependence*, 34: 29–35.

Fossey, E. (1994) *Growing Up With Alcohol*, London: Tavistock/ Routledge.

Fossey, E. and Miller, P. (1994) *Parents and alcohol education: a study in three areas*. Interim report for the Portman Group, London.

Foster, K., Wilmot, A. and Dobbs, J. (1990) *General Household Survey, 1988*, London: HMSO.

Foxcroft, D. R. and Lowe, G. (1991) 'Adolescent drinking behaviour and family socialization factors: a meta analysis', *Journal of Adolescence*, 14: 255–73.

Ghodsian, M. and Power, C. (1987) 'Alcohol consumption between the ages of 16 and 23 in Britain: a longitudinal study', *British Journal of Addiction*, 82: 175–80.

Giesbrecht, N., Gonzalez, R., Grant, M., Osterberg, E., Room, R., Rootman, I. and Towle, L. (eds) (1989) *Drinking and Casualties: Accidents, Poisonings and Violence in International Perspective*, London: Tavistock/Routledge.

Goode, E. (1972) *Drugs in American Society*, New York: Alfred A. Knopf.

Greenberg, G. S., Zucker, R. A. and Noll, R. B. (1985) *The development of cognitive structures about alcoholic beverages among preschoolers.* Paper presented at the annual meeting of the American Psychological Association, Los Angeles, CA, August.

Gronbaek, M., Deis, A., Sorensen, T., Becker, U., Borch-Johnsen, K., Muller, C., Schnohr, P. and Jensen, G. (1994) 'Influence of sex, age, body mass index and smoking on alcohol intake and mortality', *British Medical Journal*, 308: 302–6.

Ilgunas, M. (1993) *Prohibition of alcohol consumption in designated areas: an assessment.* Paper presented at conference, Alcohol: Problems and Solutions, Glasgow, 13 October.

Jahoda, G. and Cramond, J. (1972) *Children and Alcohol: A Developmental Study,* London: HMSO.

Jeffs, B. W. and Saunders, W. (1983) 'Minimising alcohol-related offences by enforcement of existing legislation', *British Journal of Addiction*, 78: 67–78.

Kalb, M. (1975) 'The myth of alcoholism prevention', *Preventive Medicine*, 4: 400–16.

Kinder, B. N., Pape, N. E. and Walfish, S. (1980) 'Drug and alcohol education programmes: a review of outcome studies', *International Journal of the Addictions*, 19: 1039–54.

Lenke, L. (1990) *Alcohol and Criminal Violence: Time Series Analyses in a Comparative Perspective,* Stockholm: Almqvist & Wiksell International.

Lister Sharp, D., (1994) 'Underage drinking in the United Kingdom since 1970: public policy, the law and adolescent drinking behaviour', *Alcohol and Alcoholism*, 29: 5–63.

Loretto, W. A. (1994a) 'Youthful drinking in Northern Ireland and Scotland: preliminary results from a comparative study', *Drugs: Education, Prevention and Policy*, 1: 143–92.

Loretto, W. A. (1994b) *Licit and Illicit Drug Use in Two Cultures: A Comparative Study of Adolescents in Scotland and Northern Ireland,* London: Harwood.

Loretto, W. A. (1994c) *Effects of income and leisure pursuits on youthful drinking.* Paper presented at 37th Scottish Alcohol Problems Symposium, Pitlochry, April.

Lowe, G. and Foxcroft, D. R. (1993) 'Young people, drinking and family life', *Alcologia*, 5: 205–9.

Marsh, A., Dobbs, J. and White, A. (1986) *Adolescent Drinking,* London: HMSO.

May, C. (1992) 'A burning issue? Adolescent alcohol use in Britain 1970–1991', *Alcohol and Alcoholism*, 27: 109–15.

May, C. (1993a) 'Control policies and youthful alcohol misuse: Effecting normative change?', *Addiction Research*, 1: 97–108.

May, C. (1993b) 'Resistance to peer pressure: an inadequate basis for alcohol education', *Health Education Research*, 8: 159–65.

May, C. (1993c) 'Young heavy drinkers: if there is a problem, is there a solution?', *Health and Social Care*, 1: 203–10.

Midanik, L. (1982) 'The validity of self-reported alcohol consumption and alcohol problems: a literature review', *British Journal of Addiction*,

77: 357–82.

Miller, P. M., Smith, G. T. and Goldman, M. S. (1990) 'Emergence of alcohol expectancies in childhood: a possible critical period', *Journal of Studies on Alcohol*, 51: 343–9.

Morgan Thomas, R. (1990) 'AIDS risks, alcohol, drugs and the sex industry: A Scottish study', in M. A. Plant (ed.) *AIDS, Drugs and Prostitution*, London: Tavistock/Routledge.

Noll, R. B. and Zucker, R. A. (1983) *Developmental findings from an alcoholic vulnerability study*. Paper presented at the annual meeting of the American Psychological Association, Anaheim, CA, August.

O' Connor, J. (1978) *The Young Drinkers*, London: Tavistock.

Osterberg, E. and Sirrka-Liisa, S. (1991) *Natural Experiments with Decreased Availability of Alcoholic Beverages: Finnish Alcohol Strikes in 1972 and 1985*, Vol. 40, Helsinki: Finnish Foundation for Alcohol Studies.

Pernanen, K. (1974) 'Validity of survey data on alcohol use', in R. J. Gibbins, Y. Israel, H. Kalant, R. E. Popham, W. Schmidt, and R. G. Smart, (eds) *Research Advances in Alcohol and Drug Problems*, Vol. 1, New York: Wiley.

Plant, M. A. (1975) *Drugtakers in an English Town*, London: Tavistock.

Plant, M. A. (1986) *Drugs in Perspective*, London: Hodder & Stoughton.

Plant, M. A. (1994a) *Reducing alcohol-related harm: a balanced and disaggregated perspective*. Paper presented at 5th International Conference on Drug-Related Harm, Toronto, Canada, 7 March.

Plant, M. A. (1994b) 'Alcohol, sex and AIDS', in L. Sherr (ed.) *AIDS and the Heterosexual Population*, Switzerland: Harwood.

Plant, M. A. and Foster, J. (1991) 'Teenagers and alcohol: results of a Scottish national survey', *Drug and Alcohol Dependence*, 28: 203–10.

Plant, M. A., Bagnall, G. and Foster, J. (1990) 'Teenage heavy drinkers: alcohol-related knowledge, beliefs, experiences, motivation and the social context of drinking' *Alcohol and Alcoholism*, 25: 691–8.

Plant, M. A., Bagnall, G., Foster, J. and Sales, J. (1991) 'Young people and drinking: results of an English national survey', *Alcohol and Alcoholism*, 25: 685–90.

Plant, M. A., Peck, D. F. and Samuel, E. (1985) *Alcohol, Drugs and School-Leavers*, London: Tavistock.

Plant, M. A. and Plant, M. L. (1992) *Risk-Takers: Alcohol, Drugs, Sex and Youth*, London: Tavistock/Routledge.

Plant, M. L. (1990) *Women and Alcohol*, Copenhagen: World Health Organization.

Plant, M. L. (1994) *Alcohol Education in Schools: A Users' Guide*, London: Portman Group.

Roberts, K. and Parsell, G. (1990) *Youth, Leisure and Alcohol: A Longitudinal Study in Four Areas*, Liverpool: University of Liverpool.

Robertson, J. A. and Plant, M. A. (1986) 'Alcohol, sex and risk of HIV infection', *Drug and Alcohol Dependence*, 22: 75–8.

Room, R. (1983) 'Alcohol and crime: behavioural aspects', in S. Kadish (ed.) *Encyclopaedia of Crime and Justice*, New York: Free Press.

Royal College of Psychiatrists (1986) *Alcohol: Our Favourite Drug*,

London: Tavistock.

Schaps, E., Dibartolo, R., Moskowitz, J, Balley, C. G. and Churgin, G. (1981) 'A review of 127 drug abuse prevention programme evaluations', *Journal of Drug Issues*, 11: 17–43.

Stall, R., McKusick, L. and Wiley, J. (1986) 'Alcohol and drug use during sexual activity and compliance with safe sex guidelines for AIDS', *Health Education Quarterly*, 13: 359–71.

Tuck, M. (1989) *Drinking and Disorder: A Study of Non-metropolitan Violence*, London: HMSO.

World Health Organisation (WHO) (1994) *Alcohol and HIV/AIDS*, Copenhagen: World Health Organisation.

Chapter 3

Alcohol and the care of older people

Larry Harrison, Jill Manthorpe and Roy Carr-Hill

INTRODUCTION

There is a major demographic shift in England and Wales, often referred to as the 'greying of the population'. By the turn of the century, about 20 per cent of the population will be over 65 years old. These demographic changes have important implications for the planning of future services, some of which have already been taken into account by government, while others are more difficult to predict. One of the elements that has not featured prominently in national discussions about service planning is the future level of alcohol-related problems. If current levels of alcohol consumption amongst the middle aged are maintained, alcohol-related morbidity will become an increasing problem among the older age groups, and current forecasts of the pattern of health and social service requirements will have to be revised.

Current estimates of the social costs of alcohol misuse (McDonnell and Maynard 1985) are not broken down by age group, but it is clear that the bulk of the criminal justice costs are generated by younger people, while most of the health care costs are incurred by older age groups. With the demographic shift, the balance of costs attributed to each of the age groups will change, as will the kinds of agencies upon which these costs fall. For example, it is likely that a greater proportion of the social costs of alcohol misuse will fall on local authority social service departments than hitherto.

In the last fifteen years clinicians have reported a relatively high prevalence of alcohol-related disabilities amongst older people (Desai and Arunachalam 1980; Jolley and Hodgson 1985; Dunne and Schipperheijn 1989). This appears to be particularly marked in hospital populations. Studies of medical and geriatric admissions over the age of 65 have shown between 5 per cent (Naik and Jones 1994) and 9 per cent (Bristow and Clare 1992) of patients drinking above the recommended levels of 21 units for men and 14 units for women: in the latter study 60 per cent of the higher risk drinkers were experiencing alcohol-related problems. Mangion *et al.* (1992) in a prospective study of 539 consecutive elderly medical admissions with a mean age of 77.3 years, identified 7.8 per cent (36 men and 6 women) as alcohol-dependent.

Similar trends have been observed by national agencies like Alcohol Concern and Help the Aged, who in the light of extensive field experience are campaigning for greater recognition of drinking problems amongst older people. Both agencies argue that alcohol consumption makes a greater contribution to morbidity amongst the over-65s than previously thought. Despite the potential importance of this issue for policies towards community care, there have been few empirical studies of the nature, range and extent of alcohol problems among older people in the UK.

One of the reasons for this neglect is that people over 65 years are seen as a low risk group for alcohol-related problems. Cross sectional surveys, in the UK, the US, and elsewhere, show that people over 65 are more likely to abstain from alcohol, and less likely to drink at high-risk levels, than those aged 18 to 59 years (Cahalan *et al.* 1969; Cahalan 1970; Knupfer 1989; Office of Population Censuses and Surveys 1990; Goddard 1991).

In the UK, risk levels for drinking are calculated in units of alcohol. A British unit of alcohol is one half pint of beer, one glass of wine or one measure of spirits: the amount of alcohol that the liver can metabolise in one hour. Based on this measure, the UK Medical Royal Colleges and the Health Education Authority have promoted the guidelines shown in Table 3.1.

Table 3.1   Guide to risk at different levels of alcohol consumption: units per week

Risk	Women	Men
Low	<15	<20
Intermediate	16–35	21–50
High	35>	50>

Table 3.2   Alcohol consumption in Great Britain by age and gender: percentage drinking above sensible levels*, 1987

	AGE COHORT			
Gender	*18–24 (%)*	*24–44 (%)*	*45–64 (%)*	*65> (%)*
Men	35	34	24	13
Women	17	14	9	4

Source: Office of Population Censuses and Surveys (1990)

* *Note:* men = over 21 units; women = over 14 units

Men drinking over 21 units and women drinking over 14 units per week are judged to be at increased risk of a range of health and social problems. Support for these estimates comes from a major longitudinal study of 12,321 British male doctors followed for 13 years (Doll *et al.* 1994). Doll *et al.* found that mortality from all causes among the over 55 year olds increased progressively with the amount drunk over 21 units.

Several national surveys have used these estimates to analyse high-risk drinking behaviours by age. Table 3.2 shows typical data for the UK, taken from the General Household Survey (GHS), a national annual study based on 10,000 households. According to the 1988 GHS only 13 per cent of men and 4 per cent of women aged 65 and over drink over the recommended 'sensible' levels, compared with 35 per cent of men, and 17 per cent per cent of women aged 18 to 24 (Office of Population Censuses and Surveys 1990: 128).

Many have argued that this reflects an inevitable decline in drinking with advancing years, possibly in response to physiological change. There are four grounds for doubting this proposition. First, the data on alcohol consumption in different age groups have been wrongly interpreted; second, variations in vulnerability have been ignored; third, the epidemiological data are inadequate; fourth, there is evidence of substantial alcohol-related morbidity amongst older people.

Inadequate consumption data

While the 1988 GHS does show relatively low consumption among the over 65s, comparisons within the GHS over a ten-year period show that self-reported rates of at-risk drinking are increasing in all age groups, including the over 65s.

Recent longitudinal research indicates that alcohol consumption does not necessarily reduce substantially with age (Glynn *et al.* 1984; Temple and Leino 1989). There appears to be a cohort effect: people who are in their 70s today grew up in the 1930s when alcohol consumption was generally much lower. Rather than being a natural consequence of ageing, the differences observed in cross-sectional surveys may reflect secular changes in drinking behaviour. If this is so, we can expect the prevalence of alcohol-related disabilities to increase in the future. UK per capita alcohol consumption has increased by over 60 per cent, in volume, over the last 30 years, and people who are in their 50s today are consuming far more alcohol than their mothers and fathers did at the same age (Robinson *et al.* 1989).

Moreover, the fact that a relatively low proportion of the over-65 age group drink heavily does not mean that the problem is insubstantial, because of the size of the older population. Table 3.3 gives estimates of the numbers of people over 65 years who are drinking at high-risk levels at any one time. The two columns on the left show the percentage of men and women in England and Wales aged over 65 years who are drinking at different risk levels. Data are derived from the Office of Population Censuses and Surveys (OPCS) dedicated drinking surveys (Goddard and Ikin 1988). Even if we adopt the more conservative estimate (1.3 per cent of older men and 0.5 per cent of older women drinking above 'safe' levels each week) many people are involved: over 4000 in Yorkshire and Humberside. If those drinking above 'sensible' levels are considered, the total rises to over 21,000 older men and 12,000 older women. Thus something like 33,000 older people may be drinking at levels which place their health at risk in any one English region – and this is without taking into account the fact that consumption in Yorkshire and Humberside is higher than the national average, which means the percentage drinking at these levels is likely to be an underestimate, nor the possibility that older people experience increased vulnerability to the effects of alcohol, which means that these risk levels may be conservative.

Table 3.3   England and Wales, and former Yorkshire Health Region:
estimated number of older people (65 and over) drinking
at high risk levels, 1990

| | ENGLAND AND WALES* | | YORKSHIRE HEALTH REGION** | | |
| | Women | Men | Women | Men | Total |
Risk	%	%	N	N	N
Exceeds sensible limit (21/14 units)	3.7	9.3	12,765	21,157	33,922
Exceeds safe limit (50/35 units)	0.5	1.3	1,725	2,957	4,682
Base (= 100%)	*541*	*440*	*345,000*	*227,500*	*572,500*

Sources:
* Percentage over 65 years drinking at different risk levels. Based on Goddard,
E. and Ikin, C. (1988) *Drinking in England and Wales in 1987*, London: HMSO.
Table 5.4.
** Population over 15, rounded. Based on Yorkshire RHA (1991), *1990 Midyear
Estimates of Population*, Harrogate: Yorkshire Regional Health Authority.

Variations in vulnerability

Even if the over-65 age group are relatively light consumers,
it would be wrong to assume they are less at risk of developing alcohol-related health problems. Current guidelines from
the Medical Royal Colleges and Health Education Authority on
'sensible' levels of alcohol consumption (under 21 units per week
for a man, 14 units for a women) may be inappropriate for older
people, who experience increased sensitivity to the effects of
alcohol (Vogel-Sprott and Chipperfield 1987). Some older people
could consume far less than the suggested risk levels and remain
vulnerable to a range of health and social problems. For example,
relatively small amounts of alcohol can cause significant central
nervous system problems, leading to confusion and falls
(Black 1990). With over three-quarters of the population over 75
receiving prescribed medication, there is also a greater risk of
cross-drug effects, resulting in harm at low levels of alcohol
consumption.

Inadequate epidemiological data

Prevalence has also been under-estimated because the methods used to identify alcohol-related problems in the older population are inadequate. There are a number of reasons why this is so, the main one being the difficulty in distinguishing between the consequences of excessive alcohol consumption and other degenerative disorders. Insomnia, depression, gastric disorders, loss of memory, cognitive impairment and tremors in older people are likely to be ascribed to dementia, Parkinson's disease and other degenerative disorders. For this reason, alcohol dependence is rarely detected when it develops late in life (Gomberg 1982; Williams 1984), while other negative consequences of excessive drinking, such as social, legal and occupational problems, are either less likely to occur after retirement or are less visible.

Hidden morbidity

The fourth reason for doubting current estimates of prevalence is that many elderly problem drinkers escape detection in the ordinary course of events. McInnes and Powell found that junior hospital doctors in New South Wales failed to identify two-thirds of ninety-nine elderly problem drinkers (McInnes and Powell 1994). Despite these difficulties, alcohol-related disorders which go unrecognised in the community are more likely to be diagnosed amongst older patients when they are admitted to hospital for other conditions, like hip fractures and metabolic bone disorders. The analysis of hospital discharge statistics in the United States shows substantial 'hidden' alcohol-related morbidity in people aged 65 years and over (Stinson et al. 1989). The age-adjusted rates for these opportunistic diagnoses amongst older people are greater than for other age groups, and point to a considerable underlying problem.

There are important cross-national differences in patterns of alcohol-related harm, however, and North American or Australian research findings cannot be assumed to apply in a British context. In order to see whether there is evidence of similar patterns in the recognition of alcohol-related morbidity amongst older people in England, Harrison and Carr-Hill (1994) undertook an analysis of the former Yorkshire regional health authority's hospital activity statistics.

Data for primary and secondary diagnoses of chronic liver disease and cirrhosis from 1975 to 1992 were obtained from the health authority and compared to population estimates for the same years. All diagnoses for chronic liver disease and cirrhosis (ICD 571) were considered, rather than diagnoses with a specific mention of alcohol (ICD 571.0–571.3), because of evidence of substantial under-reporting of specified alcoholic cirrhosis (Haberman and Weinbaum 1990), particularly for older people (Stinson et al. 1989).

In order to estimate hidden morbidity, secondary diagnoses were only considered where the primary diagnosis was not directly alcohol related (i.e. ICD 291, 303, 357.5, 425.5, 535.3, 305.0, 980). Age-adjusted rates of primary and secondary diagnoses were calculated and the data series smoothed by estimating three-year moving averages. Also, the OPCS statistics on cirrhosis mortality for England and Wales (Office of Population Censuses and Surveys 1984–93) were recalculated as age-adjusted rates per million population for the years 1975–92, and trends in these data compared to those in hospital diagnoses.

Three-year moving averages of age-adjusted rates for primary and secondary diagnoses of chronic liver disease and cirrhosis are shown in Table 3.4, and the rates for male secondary diagnoses are illustrated in Figure 3.1.

The first point to note is that while there is random fluctuation, there has been an upward shift in both primary and secondary diagnoses for all age groups, which is more marked for secondary diagnoses. Indeed the test for trends using the Pearson correlation coefficient for the different age–sex groups for both primary and secondary diagnoses, given in Table 3.5, makes this clear: they are most often significant for secondary diagnoses among males.

The overall increase in both primary and secondary diagnoses for cirrhosis is reflected in the rise in cirrhosis mortality nationally. Figure 3.2 shows the trend in mortality for England and Wales by age for the years 1975–1992.

Finally, it can be seen that in all age groups, the rates for secondary diagnoses are substantial, relative to the rates for primary diagnoses, and that the ratio of secondary to primary diagnosis is highest for those aged 65 years and over. The percentage of 'hidden morbidity' is shown in Figure 3.3 which makes the point more graphically. It looks as if there might have been a slight upward shift for males, although this is not statistically significant.

Table 3.4 Chronic liver disease and cirrhosis (ICD9–571) in the Yorkshire region: rates of primary and secondary diagnosis by age, 1975–1991 (3 year rolling averages)

Men	Primary diagnosis			Secondary diagnosis		
	25–44	45–64	65+	25–44	45–64	65+
1977	7.54	27.31	19.4	1.77	12.75	16.24
1978	9.29	29.26	23.56	2.56	12.48	15.9
1979	10.36	28.56	24.32	2.75	12.02	14.22
1980	11.08	30.46	26.15	3.59	12.11	15.43
1981	11.63	30.44	26.51	2.93	13.8	18.89
1982	11.57	33.52	26.99	3.13	12.83	21.03
1983	12.29	34.15	31.06	3.8	14.94	19.52
1984	11.4	31.97	32.86	4.62	14.44	17.29
1985	10.93	29.24	35.62	4.85	15.39	17.25
1986	9.82	27.31	34.77	3.62	14.82	19.85
1987	8.58	26.75	31.7	3.94	16.47	24.49
1988	8.34	26.09	26.4	5.36	19.39	29.87
1989	11.01	28.22	26.22	6.79	22.59	35.25
1990	11.77	30.36	28.73	8.65	24.76	33.49
1991	13.47	33.79	36.49	7.59	26.11	35.82

Women	Primary diagnosis			Secondary diagnosis		
	25–44	45–64	65+	25–44	45–64	65+
1977	3.84	24.11	23.83	1.61	8.06	14.71
1978	5.04	23.62	20.41	1.50	9.85	13.17
1979	4.24	24.50	18.68	1.86	9.41	12.72
1980	4.57	26.42	16.97	2.06	9.44	11.38
1981	5.78	28.61	18.64	3.15	9.46	12.70
1982	7.41	27.39	21.38	3.56	10.01	11.08
1983	7.73	26.03	24.44	3.11	10.68	10.12
1984	7.81	25.40	22.99	2.40	10.09	9.37
1985	6.16	26.31	23.20	1.66	8.62	10.97
1986	6.54	25.63	21.09	1.77	7.56	12.11
1987	5.41	25.75	23.47	1.91	9.12	14.21
1988	5.40	24.93	22.16	2.19	12.64	15.63
1989	7.08	25.94	23.09	3.55	13.73	17.87
1990	8.41	26.32	23.07	4.07	15.35	18.84
1991	9.71	29.24	25.89	5.21	18.28	21.87

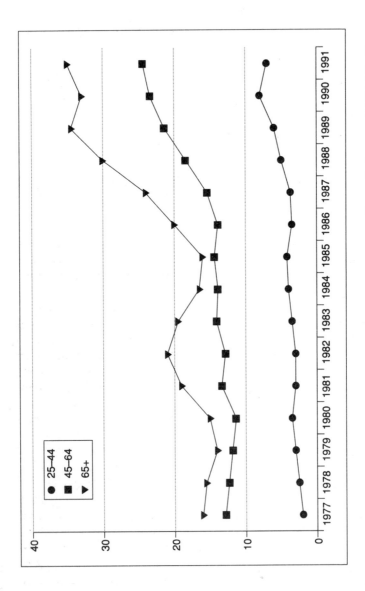

Figure 3.1 Chronic liver disease and cirrhosis: male rates of secondary diagnosis by age (1977–91). Three year rolling averages.

Table 3.5 Liver cirrhosis primary and secondary diagnosis; Pearson correlation coefficient of rates against years

	MALES		FEMALES	
Age	Primary	Secondary	Primary	Secondary
25–44	0.18	0.89**	0.52*	0.58*
45–64	−0.05	0.90**	0.48	0.70**
65+	0.63*	0.87**	0.36	0.51
Total	0.9	0.90**	0.24	0.67**

Notes: *p < 0.05; **p < 0.01

A number of caveats are necessary in relation to the findings on secular trends. First, the pre-1985 data are derived from the Hospital In Patient Enquiry (HIPE), and the post-1985 data from the Hospital Episodes Statistics (HES). The move from HIPE to HES may have led to some double counting. Testing for the impact of HES did not show any major discontinuity, however, and the observed upward trend is also reflected in the national mortality figures.

Second, many clinicians will be suspicious of any analysis of officially recorded statistics like the HES because of their knowledge of the way in which such data are obtained. While there may be a degree of under-reporting in the HES, which would make it unreliable for estimating prevalence, the errors are likely to be consistent and in the same direction, and therefore the trends within the data are likely to hold.

Third, the analysis is based on data for the former York-shire Health Region, which has one of the highest levels of alcohol consumption in the United Kingdom (Office of Population Censuses and Surveys 1992). It is possible – indeed likely – that other regions have lower levels of alcohol-related problems among the over 65s, since alcohol-related hospitalisa-tions for older people have been shown to be strongly corre-lated with regional per capita consumption in the United States (Adams *et al.* 1993). Nevertheless, the rise observed in York-shire in primary and secondary diagnoses for all age groups, but particularly for the over 65s, mirrors the rise in national age-adjusted rates of cirrhosis mortality over the same period.

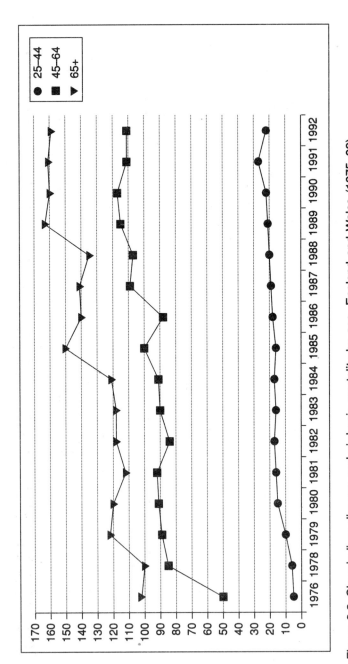

Figure 3.2 Chronic liver disease and cirrhosis mortality by age, England and Wales (1975–92).

Source: calculated from OPCS (1976–93).

Note: rates of death (ICD 571) per million population in each cohort

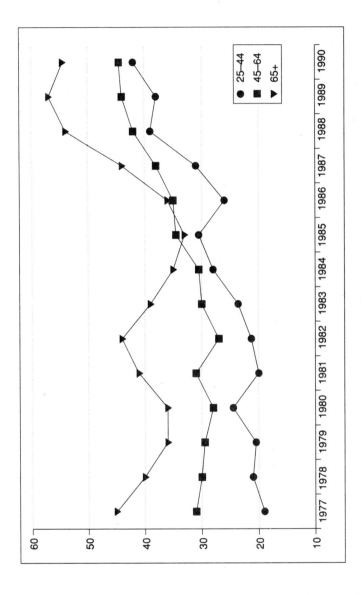

Figure 3.3 Secondary diagnosis of chronic liver disease and cirrhosis among men in Yorkshire as a percentage of all cirrhosis diagnoses, by age (1977–91). Three year rolling averages

Despite the limitations of hospital activity statistics for epidemiological studies over time there is one clear message: those aged
65 years and over in the Yorkshire region are much more likely
than younger patients to receive a secondary diagnosis of chronic
liver disease and cirrhosis when admitted to hospital for a diagnosis which is not obviously alcohol-related. There is no reason
to suppose that the move from HIPE to HES would affect this,
nor that the ability of hospital doctors in Yorkshire to identify
cirrhosis is markedly different from their colleagues elsewhere.

It is possible that much of this morbidity would have gone unde-
tected in the absence of hospitalisation for the primary diagnosis.
Further investigation would be needed to establish whether the
same holds true for other alcohol-related diagnoses, but the age-
related effect observed here supports the hypothesis that there is
substantial unrecognised alcohol-related morbidity among older
people in the community.

IMPLICATIONS FOR SERVICES

Such findings have particular relevance for welfare professionals
in the area of care management and purchasing or provision of
services. In this section we shall explore these using a care management framework (Orme and Glastonbury 1993), acknowledging
that local implementation of the NHS and Community Care Act
1990 has resulted in a host of geographical variations.

The essence of care management is that it is a service provided
to people with long-term care needs. As Challis notes (1994) it
comprises a generally agreed set of core tasks – case finding and
screening; assessment; care planning; implementation and monitoring. However, it is more than a set of processes, since the care
manager's role often involves advocacy to some extent and the
integration of care from a variety of formal and informal networks
(Challis 1994: 62). Previous structures which existed to respond
to client characteristics rarely delivered innovative, flexible and
quality services – particularly in respect of people with multiple
social and health care needs of a long-term or indeterminate
nature.

The needs of a minority of older people have always been at
the heart of care management, particularly those without financial resources or intensive human support networks and who are
variously disabled by long-standing health problems, mental or

physical illness or accumulated disabilities. It is against this background that care management has evolved as a major procedural mechanism to implement the NHS and Community Care Act 1990.

Case finding and screening

Richardson (1995: 241), in an attempt to introduce a jargon-free language of care management, refers to this task as, 'identifying specific individuals for attention'. As we illustrated earlier there is a general lack of appreciation that older people may have alcohol problems and few community care plans see them as a group that needs identification by virtue of their alcohol-related problems.

Many community care plans are written on the basis of established client groups, and while 80 per cent of a sample of plans for 1993–94 (Hardy *et al.* 1993) included people who misuse drugs and/or alcohol, the separation of this group from other equally distinctive categories such as older people can artificially distance the two.

The policy debate, evident in other aspects of gerontology, is whether older people are a separate group, by virtue of their chronological age, or whether it is ageist to look at the predominant need or problem. In essence we need to assess whether older people with alcohol-related problems should be encapsulated within services for older people or whether services for people with alcohol problems should include adults of all ages.

This debate over integration versus segregation has often been left aside as services have developed on largely incremental lines and are moulded to a great extent by local politics, professional interests, tradition and even personalities. As Chapter 8 shows, alcohol services have been criticised for designing services for men, and in particular white men of working age. One of the challenges of the demographic shift of the population to alcohol services will be their ability to mirror such changes, in particular relating to an older age profile of service users, a number of whom might be women and for whom employment or family support is less likely.

In this – the first broad area of care management – the information gap is highlighted concerning older people with alcohol problems. This will affect priority given to developing services and even in making optimum use of existing services. Few authorities are in a position to estimate numbers involved and to design a list of relevant information about local contacts or resources. Information held by one service is not readily available to other purchasers or providers.

An early report on the development of care management arrangements in seven local authorities notes that overall the authorities were still struggling with:

a. the speed of response
b. the level of assessment
c. priority access to resources
d. access to particular services

(Department of Health 1994: 30)

It is the latter two elements that govern access to the funding released by care management services, but for older people with alcohol problems the debate has not really started about priorities or which particular access routes are appropriate.

Lastly, in this area, is a need to reflect on one of the over-arching policy themes of the Department of Health. In the White Paper *Caring for People* emphasis is put on:

promoting positive and healthy lifestyles among all age groups through health education and the development of effective health surveillance and screening programmes and so reducing as far as possible the need for in-patient and residential care

(1989: para 2.12: 11)

This aspect of community care has largely been forgotten. Local authorities have in a few cases embarked upon 'Healthy Cities' initiatives or other collaborative public health measures, but these have largely been outwith their community care arrangements and have led to services that appear less able to prevent problems arising than to deal with resultant crises. One of the challenges for policy-makers will be how to translate these other objectives into action.

Assessment

The translation of adult services from resource-led to needs-led services was seen as one of the key aspects of implementing the objectives set out in *Caring for People*. In order to determine appropriate, individualised and preferred services various government recommendations have been issued, outlining who should be involved in the assessment process, the input of user and carer(s), the need to establish and publicise criteria and details of what information should be included and how it should be verified. Initial research suggests that this procedural guidance has had certain problems – it leads to descriptive rather than analytical material; proformas are complex and lengthy; information may not be shared (Department of Health 1994).

What seems to be developing in response to these problems is specialist assessment documentation and gradation of assessment into simple, specialist and comprehensive or multi-disciplinary types (Department of Health 1994: 9).

For older people with suspected alcohol-related problems assessment needs to be sensitive to the needs of the person as a whole. Accurate description will assist in distinguishing the person with problems from those who may have conditions mimicking alcohol-related disorder as discussed earlier. Assessment is not simply verbal communication, but for the social worker will include all the senses – seeing whether self-neglect might be a concern, or loss of weight, smelling alcohol or signs of self-neglect, hearing the story of a person's typical day or how they are 'managing'. For many assessment visits, a proforma may assist in collecting data, but may inhibit asking about biographical details, life histories and hopes or fears about loss, disability or death.

Many social workers are reluctant to ask for details of people's finances (Deere 1994) but suspected alcohol problems may mean that an older person is in significant debt or is unable to provide for necessities. Where a significant element of mental confusion exists, it may be appropriate to consider protecting a person's finances through the Benefits Agency or Court of Protection or Enduring Power of Attorney (if arranged early).

We drew attention earlier to the problems that may arise in determining alcohol-related problems among older people. For social workers and others working in community care the problems may be slow to develop and may not show up in initial assessment. There may be difficulties in communicating concerns across the wide range of services involved – particularly now the pluralist basis for community care may mean involvement from informal carers, voluntary groups, local authorities, Health Trusts, not-for-profit and commercial sectors, the primary health care team (perhaps fund-holding) and services such as housing providers, libraries, churches, and so on, whose primary purpose is not community care delivery.

To address such coordination problems, a number of older people, having been assessed as being in need of significant personal and/or social care, will have the services of a named care manager. Such workers, with a limited but intensive caseload may well be able to ensure a further reassessment if alcohol problems are uncovered or develop. This of course depends on their ability to see that alcohol may be a factor to consider, and on their knowledge of sources of help and advice.

Implementing the care package

In more expansionist definitions of community care, care packages may result in any service at whatever level and may include residential care, day services, domiciliary support or respite care. In this section the focus will be on one particular issue arising from care management work with older people for whom there is concern that their alcohol intake is damaging their health. It is in the context of consumerist theories that are an integral part of community care philosophy, determining whether the recipient of services has control or is 'empowered' (see Means and Smith 1994 for a full discussion). Many of the debates in this area fail to address the control functions of social work and rarely give examples based on practice. However, the instance of an older person who, as part of the care package of domestic assistance, wishes to purchase alcohol on a regular basis, throws up some of the dilemmas of putting empowerment into practice.

Case example:
Mr. A is housebound and lives alone. He asks his domestic assistant (paid for by Social Services who recoup Mr A's attendance allowance) to make regular purchases of beer. The house is cold and unkempt and Mr A has poor personal hygiene. He clearly drinks several pints of beer daily and is sometimes 'tipsy' according to the domestic assistant, Mrs B. She wants to know if she can stop buying Mr A his beer and asks his care manager.

There are three 'actors' in this case example and it might be useful for training purposes to discuss the perspective of each. The issues for Mrs B are that she fears money is being spent on beer, not heat nor food and that 'it can't be good' for Mr A to drink so much. She believes that stopping or limiting Mr A's drinking would benefit him, but might make him angry with her. She wants guidance from the care manager.

This social worker has assessed Mr B as needing significant help with tasks of daily living. She knows that he lives in poor circumstances and has a limited social life, but that he does not want to be 'tidy' or to go out to a day centre. She has put together a care package that relies on Mrs B to call in daily to do housework, shopping and some food preparation. From her interviews with Mr A she recalls how difficult it was to get him to accept any assistance.

Mr A is our notional consumer. He 'pays' for Mrs B to provide domestic help and feels that she should do what he wants. He feels it is none of her business how he spends his money and that she is a 'bossy young woman'.

There are three potential conflicts here, in a situation that may well be complicated by the presence of Mr A's doctor, any relatives and the employer of Mrs B (who may be delivering home care through a contract with an independent agency). For the care manager, good practice would involve strategies that would:

- raise the issue with Mr B so that he could be included in the discussion;
- discuss the risks involved with Mr B and Mrs A and put them into perspective and some order of priority.
- see if Mr B's drinking is associated with loneliness or an unresolved mental health problem, such as depression.

Many older problem drinkers appear socially isolated but the relationship between heavy alcohol consumption and links to social networks is unclear. A study of older men in the Swedish city of Malmö (Hanson 1994) indicated that it was not possible to tell if social isolation influences the drinking of alcohol, or if alcohol causes social isolation. Hanson also points out that some social networks may exacerbate alcohol consumption. He calls for longitudinal research to test the effectiveness of intervention programmes.

Frogatt (1990) notes that the support network for older people may be particularly important in helping those with alcohol-related problems. One crucial role for a care manager may lie in working on reestablishing such a network or setting up new links that can have meaning or provide some scope for the older person to feel less isolated or to have greater self-esteem. Such networking may involve far wider contacts than those involved in seeking care or practical social assistance and can include involvement in voluntary or pressure groups activities, neighbourhood contacts, taking up hobbies, new skills or reestablishing contact with religious bodies, occupational or retirement groups or ex-service organisations.

Most importantly, the care manager should be able to draw on existing networks of professional advice and support that will give him or her the benefit of the specialist services. Both workers with older people and older people themselves need to challenge marginalisation within specialist services that concentrate on younger people.

Residential care

A number of older people's care packages will include living in residential or nursing homes, on a permanent basis or for rehabilitation or respite purposes. The workhouse image which lingers in many people's minds, particularly if they are elderly, was bound up with restricted diets and unstimulating activities in which choice and resources were limited. The Wagner Committee noted that choice, independence, dignity and privacy should be hallmarks of residential life (Wagner *et al.* 1988), and one of the criteria for assessing whether these values are adhered to in a residential home is the existence of 'rules about smoking and alcohol which take account of dignity of consumers and others' (Social Services Inspectorate 1989: 58). The provision of alcohol or choice about its availability has become a benchmark to suggest positive features of residential care.

The availability of alcohol is generally regarded in a positive light by older residents themselves. In a research project which asked older people to assess what was important to them in a residential home, one-third of men and one-quarter of women mentioned alcoholic beverages (Willcocks *et al.* 1987). This indicates that while it is not essential, for a number of older people a normal environment would include the provision of alcohol. Service providers need to consider how these demands are best met, while not exacerbating the risks from alcohol consumption faced by older people.

This chapter has shown that the extent of alcohol-related problems among older people has been under-estimated, and demographic change means that there are likely to be many more older people with drinking problems in the years to come. We have outlined some of the difficulties this will pose for community care and suggested how the health and personal social services might respond.

REFERENCES

Adams, W. L., Yuan, Z., Barboriak, J. J. and Rimm, A. A. (1993) 'Alcohol-related hospitalisations of elderly people: prevalence and geographical location in the United States', *Journal of the American Medical Association*, 270: 1222–5.

Aitken, L. (1995) *Ageing*, New York: Sage.

Black, D. (1990) 'Changing patterns and consequences of alcohol abuse in old age', *Geriatric Medicine*, (January): 19–20.

Bristow, M. F. and Clare, A. W. (1992) 'Prevalence and characteristics of at-risk drinkers among elderly acute medical in-patients', *British Journal of Addiction*, 87(2): 291–4.

Cahalan, D. (1970) *Problem Drinkers: A National Survey*, San Francisco, CA: Jossey-Bass.

Cahalan, D., Cisin, I. H. and Crossley, H. M. (1969) *American Drinking Practices: A National Study of Drinking Behavior and Attitudes*, New Brunswick, NJ: Rutgers Center for Alcohol Studies.

Challis, D. (1994) 'Care Management' in N. Malin (ed.) *Implementing Community Care*, Buckingham: Open University Press.

Deere, J. (1994) 'Financial Skills, First Steps', *Care Plan*, 1 Sept., 1: 28–9.

Department of Health (1989) *Caring for People Community Care in the Next Decade and Beyond*, Cm. 849, London: HMSO.

Department of Health (1992) *Health of the Nation: A Strategy for Health in England*, London: HMSO.

Department of Health (1994) *Implementing Community Care: Care Management*, London: Department of Health.

Desai, H. and Arunachalam, S. (1980) 'When age plus alcoholism can be misleading', *Geriatric Medicine*, June: 11–4.

Doll, R., Peto, R., Hall, E., Wheatley, K. and Gray, R. (1994) 'Mortality in relation to consumption of alcohol: 13 years' observations on male British doctors', *British Medical Journal*, 309: 911–8.

Dunne, F. J. and Schipperheijn, J. A. M. (1989) 'Alcohol and the Elderly', *British Medical Journal*, 298(6689): 1660–1.

Frogatt, A. (1990) *Family Work with Elderly People*, London: BASW/ Macmillan.

Glynn, R. L., Bouchard, G. R., LoCastro, J. S. and Hermos, J. A. (1984) 'Changes in alcohol consumption behaviors among men in the Normative Aging Study', in G. Maddox, L. N. Robins and N. Rosenberg (eds) *Nature and Extent of Alcohol Problems Among the*

Elderly, Research Monograph No. 14. DHHS Pub. No. (ADM) 84–1321 Washington, DC: Government Printing Office.

Goddard, E. (1991) *Drinking in England and Wales in the late 1980s*, London: HMSO.

Goddard, E. and Ikin, C. (1988) *Drinking in England and Wales in 1987*, London: HMSO.

Gomberg, E. (1982) 'Alcohol use and problems among the elderly', in National Institute on Alcohol Abuse and Alcoholism (ed.) *Alcohol and Health Monograph 4*, Washington, DC: US Government Printing Office.

Haberman, P. W. and Weinbaum, D. F. (1990) 'Liver cirrhosis with and without mention of alcohol as cause of death', *British Journal of Addiction*, 85(2): 217–22.

Hanson, B. (1994) 'Social network, social support and heavy drinking in elderly men: a population study of men born in 1914 in Malmö, Sweden', *Addiction*, 89: 725–32.

Hardy, B., Wistow, G. and Leedham, I. (1993) *Analysis of a Sample of English Community Care Plans 1993/4*, Leeds: Nuffield Institute for Health/Department of Health.

Harrison, L. and Carr-Hill, R. (1994) *Alcohol and Older People: Estimating the 'Dark Figure' of Unrecognised Morbidity*, Hull: University of Hull.

Jacyk, J., Tabisz, E. and Badger, M. (1991) 'Chemical dependency in the elderly: identification phase', *Canadian Journal of Ageing*, 10 (1): 10–17.

Jolley, D. and Hodgson, S. (1985) 'Alcoholism in the elderly: a tale of women and our times', *Recent Advances in Geriatric Medicine*, 3: 113–22.

Knupfer, G. (1989) 'The prevalence in various social groups of eight different drinking patterns', *British Journal of Addiction*, 84(11): 1305–18.

Mangion, D. M., Platt, J. S. and Syam, V. (1992) 'Alcohol and acute medical admission of elderly people', *Age and Aging*, 21: 362–7.

McDonnell, R. and Maynard, A. (1985) 'The costs of alcohol misuse', *British Journal of Addiction*, 80: 27–36.

McInnes, E. and Powell, J. (1994) 'Drug and alcohol referrals: are elderly substance abuse diagnoses and referrals being missed?', *British Medical Journal*, 308(6926): 444–6.

Means, R. and Smith, R. (1994) *Community Care: Policy and Practice*, London: Macmillan.

Naik, P. C. and Jones, R. G. (1994) 'Alcohol histories taken from elderly people on admission', *British Medical Journal*, 308(6923): 248.

Office of Population Censuses and Surveys (1984–93) *Mortality Statistics: Cause*, London: HMSO.

Office of Population Censuses and Surveys (1990) *General Household Survey 1988*, London: HMSO.

Office of Population Censuses and Surveys (1992) *General Household Survey 1990*, London: HMSO.

Orme, J. and Glastonbury, B. (1993) *Care Management*, London: Macmillan.

Richardson, A. (1995) 'Care management' in N. Malin (ed.) *Services for People with Learning Disabilities*, London: Routledge.

Robinson, D., Maynard, A. and Chester, R., (eds) (1989) *Controlling Legal Addictions*, London: Macmillan.

Social Services Inspectorate (1989) *Homes Are For Living In*, London: Department of Health.

Stinson, F. S., Dufour, M. C. and Bertolucci, D. (1989) 'Epidemiologic Bulletin No. 20: alcohol-related morbidity in the aging population', *Alcohol Health and Research World*, 13(1): 80–7.

Temple, M. T. and Leino, V. (1989) 'Long-term outcomes of drinking: a 20 year longitudinal study of men', *British Journal of Addiction*, 84(8): 889–99.

Turner, G., Wilson, P., Ward, G., James, S., and Legg, E. (1990) 'What proportion of falls in elderly people who present to hospital are related to alcohol drinking?' *Care of the Elderly*, 2 (10): 413–4.

Vetter, N., Lewis, P. and Charny, M. (1990) 'Lifestyle and the elderly', *Health Education Journal*, 49 (2): 76–9.

Vogel-Sprott, M. and Chipperfield, B. (1987) 'Family history of problem drinking among young male social drinkers: behavioural effects of alcohol', *Journal of Studies on Alcohol*, 48: 430–6.

Wagner, J., and National Institute for Social Work (1988) *Residential Care: A Positive Choice, Report of the Independent Review of Residential Care*, London: HMSO.

Willcocks, D., Peace, S., and Kellaher, L. (1987) *Private Lives in Public Places*, London: Tavistock.

Williams, M. (1984) 'Alcohol and the elderly: an overview', *Alcohol Health and Research World*, 8(3): 3–9.

Chapter 4

People with learning disabilities: alcohol and ordinary lives

Jill Manthorpe

INTRODUCTION

This chapter looks at the role of alcohol in the lives of people with learning disabilities, in an age when the consumption of alcohol almost represents a badge of citizenship. Such citizenship and the very notion of adult status has long been denied to many people with learning disabilities. Consuming alcohol is a risk, in the true sense of the word, meaning that it is composed of possible benefits and dangers (see Alaszewski and Manthorpe 1991) and people with learning disabilities have been 'protected' from socially undesirable risks by a variety of policies and care practices. Community care, and the closure of long-stay mental handicap hospitals in particular, challenge this protective, paternalist environment.

This chapter looks at alcohol consumption in a broad sense, and is keen to avoid a social pathology model which sees alcohol solely as a problem in which professionals ought to intervene and adopt new controls. It starts with an examination of alcohol consumption as part of ordinary life, particularly when associated with leisure. The literature here refers to the positive associations of the 'pub' or public house and so has a generally British or Irish context. It should be remembered though that going to the pub need not necessarily equate with drinking alcohol: it is a leisure activity that can include soft drinks, active games participation and, increasingly, meals.

Positive associations are qualified however by the experiences of some people who find pub life unstimulating or so artificially constructed that the value of its role as an ordinary life activity is highly suspect. For others, pubs and their associations are unwelcome and threatening. We describe how one social education project uses pub life as part of an educational process for a group of young men in their transition to adult status.

The next section looks at specific implications for community care services: namely integrating alcohol education into individual learning about diet and nutrition generally and raising awareness about the possible interaction of medication and alcohol. The subject of foetal alcohol syndrome is also raised in this section, as well as help for people with alcohol-related problems.

Lastly this chapter draws attention to the need for community care services to consider staff policies in this area, where staff's role often means treading a delicate path between controlling vulnerable adults' lives and allowing them to behave in ways which might be harmful to themselves or others. Staff policies also need to consider issues such as whether staff should be allowed to consume alcohol at work.

Discussions about alcohol and people with learning disabilities reveal a general lack of interest in alcohol as part and parcel of ordinary life. Useful exercises may be conducted in life history work to explore the patterns in the lives of the majority of people with disabilities who are not linked to institutions. Unfortunately there are few life-history documents or autobiographies as yet (though Atkinson 1994 offers a useful starter). Instead we have to turn to accounts of the lives of people with learning disabilities written for other purposes.

Booth and Booth (1994) offer such an opportunity in some of their interviews with parents who have learning disabilities. The lives of their respondents are rich in data, particularly around issues of suspected child abuse and neglect of the parent's need. They also reveal that many 'ordinary lives', despite a deal of poverty and deprivation, often involve community presence in pubs, working men's clubs, parties and socialising. In the account of the life of Rosie Spencer, a poignant account of the end of the research is marked by a final outing for researcher and respondent:

> We find a warm and cosy pub, although it is virtually empty. Rosie has a small beer and some crisps. We talk for over an hour and Rosie follows with a large cream sherry. We celebrate.
>
> (Booth and Booth 1994: 108)

Nowhere is the 'ordinary life' aspect of going to a pub more simply and effectively portrayed. Alcohol, we are given to understand, links both subject of research and researcher across their differences in life experiences, though interestingly we only see what Rosie drinks and eats. There is no suggestion that either of them needs educating or has problems.

For people with learning disabilities the ability to visit 'the pub' is seen in contrast to institutional services which can be inflexible and building-based. Wright *et al.* (1994), for example, suggest that a service brokerage system, enhancing the consumer power of care management, might include:

> flexible and mobile staff teams, to enable and support people to take advantage of community resources and opportunities, from going to the pub with friends to undertaking full-time employment.
>
> (1994: 43)

They term this 'getting alongside' support which enables people to participate in community activities. They argue that 'enabling the person to go to the pub' is given as an example typical of community participation which has 'massive potential benefits for users and could help to remove attitudinal barriers in society as a whole' (ibid.: 123).

Alcohol and leisure

Cahill (1994: 157) notes that television, alcohol, tobacco, sex and gambling are the most popular leisure activities reported by British adults currently. He remarks that many are organised by commercial or profit-making interests. Additionally many people attend other organised leisure events where alcohol may be widely available, even if the organisation is totally informal such as parties, or semi-formal such as fund-raising events run by local voluntary groups.

Clearly leisure is still a highly gendered and age-stratified activity. It is also a product of tradition, with the male use of the public house often given as a classic response to harsh manual work (Cahill 1994: 154). The local geography of an area may determine which venues are defined as 'male space' or more recently have become significant locations for those with particular sexual orientations, lifestyles (e.g. students) or occupations (e.g. market traders, armed forces, etc.). The concept of the 'local' (public house) is therefore highly variable. It may exist or it may not and what does exist may change. This unpredictability should not surprise anyone working in community care but it does mean support structures need to be clearly understood and related to their social context. Tyne's example of Ted (a man with learning disabilities) notes that his support included a friend 'who has known Ted for many years [and who] calls regularly at their local pub' (1992: 36). In this case both men appear to find the environment amenable, and for Ted it appears to score highly in the five accomplishments mentioned below. At the other extreme Brown and Smith (1992: 167) acknowledge that there may be some pubs who ask people with disabilities to leave and that these should be actively challenged and widely boycotted.

For workers in community care services, knowledge of the resources of a local area needs to include the type of facilities that may be part of service users' lives. This is clearly relevant to the philosophical values of normalisation so that having a drink or a meal in a local pub serves a number of functions, such as community presence, participation, making choices, developing competence and enhancing respect. These 'five accomplishments', discussed in the context of the development of normalisation (Emerson 1992: 14) are overwhelmingly positive in tone. Yet when applied to alcohol consumption they reveal how superficial interpretations of normalisation have often ignored cultural and other factors of social stratification. For example, reactions to drinking of alcohol vary considerably in terms of respect. For some individuals, or groups with particular religious or moral beliefs, it is an activity to be condemned. For others, this rather blanket disapproval is applied to women, for example, or women of certain ages or marital status.

Sensitivity to cultural factors is then a key feature of work in community care for service users. For some service users there will be dilemmas in balancing their own choice of activities against pressures from others. Staff have to empower users to manage such tensions and to articulate their problems. At the moment such work is rather confined to issues of sexuality – Cahill's other leisure areas are largely ignored.

Discussions about the role of alcohol in leisure are generally based outwith the domestic context – with public houses still predominant as a cultural image. This view ignores both the drinking of alcohol in restaurants, the consumption of alcohol at home (whether home is a small or large unit) and the common practice of home production of alcoholic drinks ('home-brewed beer or wine'). For people with learning disabilities these aspects of social life are part of their hidden lives. We can predict however that much will be dependent on staff views, where accommodation has major staff support, or individuals' interests and perhaps assistance from family or friends. Shearer's reference to wine-making (1986: 159) is one of the few reports to include this activity as part of leisure for people with learning disabilities.

There are many positive aspects of going to the pub. It is a commonly accepted, valued activity. In many ways it stands as an image of 'normal' or 'ordinary' life for it is neither segregated nor organised. None the less, going to the pub need not be the height of anyone's social expectations: for many people it is not enough and for some, particular local circumstances or individual preferences make the pub less attractive. Shearer (1986) describes how one young person involved in the Outreach project for Jewish Youth in Greater Manchester found life fairly predictable: 'We only ever went out to the pub. Now you can do your own things. It's much better' (1986: 162).

In terms of professional practice such a view warns that assessment of individuals' needs to be broadly based and to understand that what is positive for one person may be constricting or boring for another.

Within residential care the pub may be used as an aspect of community life, spanning institutional and domestic environments, or maintaining community links. On the other hand it can be used as a 'reward' or 'treat', removing choice over behaviour and implicitly infantilising the residents. McCormack's description of the voluntary-sector residential home, Chadwick House (anonymised), conveys this sense well, and despite the date of her research (1979) such attitudes may well persist. One resident, Harry, describes how his view of 'freedom' would be to be able to go to the pub alone. It appears that occasional visits to the pub are made with members of staff. Notably, McCormack reports (without comment): 'Birthday girls and boys have the choice of a trip to the pub with a few friends or a disco-session in the lounge' (McCormack 1979: 177). In this home most residents go to bed at 9 p.m.

The case of Jerry, for example, a Black British man in his 40s with Down's syndrome, illustrates that going to the pub might be a fairly regular and routine activity, but in the company of people (residents and staff) whom he is with all week, it is not an opportunity to meet other people, particularly those from his original Jamaican community. A Central Council for Education and Training in Social Work (CCETSW) training manual (Bano *et al.* 1993) comments that Jerry lives his life according to the norms of a White Englishman:

> He attends an Adult Training Centre five days a week and has a very limited social life mainly centring on a visit to the pub with his fellow residents and members of staff.
>
> (1993: 49)

While staff may see his leisure time as spent appropriately, the criticism implied in the CCETSW manual suggests that Jerry may need to have the choice of broader social contacts – going to pubs if this is what he likes but in the company of others of Jamaican backgrounds perhaps where music, games and activities may reflect different preferences.

Living with alcohol

Much of this chapter has looked at the social context of alcohol consumption in a positive light. However, like other individuals, people with learning disabilities may find that increased vulnerability puts them at risk from others who abuse alcohol or have other dependencies. Research into the abuse and mistreatment of older people by family members shows that alcohol dependence is a clear risk factor (Wolf 1990) among perpetrators of physical, psychological and financial abuse.

This subject arises in work with people with learning disabilities. For some the abuse is not physical but part of a context of psychological harm and distress. Gilbert (1995), for example, describes how Margaret Adams' control over her own life was undermined by her father. Having recently made her give up her holiday plans her father took Margaret to the dog races:

> Following this he met some friends at the pub and totally ignored Margaret, and after getting quite drunk he invited his friends back to the house for a nightcap and a fish supper.

... Then, as they were all drinking, the TV was switched on for an 'adult' film. In front of all these people Mr Adams sent Margaret to bed.

(1995: 127)

In this example, while the effect of alcohol is not simplistically linked to violence or abuse, it forms an undercurrent of sexual threat which is clearly a prominent cultural association with alcohol, particularly for women.

Living with family members who have problems with alcohol may also affect the socialisation of people with learning disabilities with regard to appropriate patterns of alcohol consumption. It is hard for professional workers to conduct education programmes about health issues when contradictory and confusing messages may be received. For example, a person who is learning about sensible eating at an educational centre may return home to a family where other members are behaving in ways that would not be deemed sensible, such as missing meals, spending money on alcohol rather than food or eating 'junk' food.

Behavioural techniques are behind many of the teaching programmes that operate in the area of education of people with learning disabilities. However, in line with historical concern about aspects of learning disabilities far more attention is given to sexuality and personal relationships than to education about sensible drinking. Behind such programmes as do exist there are attempts to shape sequences of behaviour in which appropriate patterns are learned. Thus a person might be encouraged to accept a personal limit to alcohol consumption (e.g. two pints of beer), and then could be assisted both to 'say no' to further alcohol and also to maintain sociability by moving to soft drinks. For people whose medication or physical condition make alcohol inadvisable, strategies to maintain self-respect could be learned and practised in realistic settings. The example of peers (rather than staff) might be used to reinforce patterns; if not alternative models of behaviour will have to be devised.

Currently such work is often unfocused in respect of alcohol education. Examples of refusing or accepting an alcoholic drink are used instead as illustrations of confidence building or assertiveness as we shall see below.

Alcohol and adulthood

The transition from childhood to adulthood has various markers in contemporary Western society but for many people there are important milestones such as being legally permitted to drive, engage in sexual activity with others, or purchase tobacco or alcohol.

All of these are potentially difficult for young people with learning disabilities. In relation to alcohol there are external factors which may restrict individuals' opportunities to join their peers in common social activities, such as going to the pub. First, many young people with learning disabilities have limited incomes as formal and informal employment opportunities are restricted. They are not alone in this, but many do not have control over their benefits or grants. Second, many young people with learning disabilities live at home with their parents in a child/parent relationship where a measure of parental control is exercised to protect the younger person. Third, as Richardson and Ritchie (1989) illustrate in their study of friendship patterns, young people with learning disabilities often find it difficult to become friends with a person without disabilities. Segregated education means neighbourhood peer relationships may not have evolved. A young adult with learning disabilities may therefore have few friends in the community or locality, may have few resources to spend or to use to develop a fashionable image with the necessary consumer labels, and may feel under pressure to remain involved in family-centred rather than peer-group activities.

Hazelhurst (1990) describes a group work project that lasted two years involving young men with learning disabilities in London. In total, ten young men with moderate learning disabilities, referred from a variety of agencies, attended the group with the purpose of developing their social lives and through that their communication skills.

The first in a list of tasks identified by the group members as important markers of adult status, was: 'going into a pub, buying a drink and acting sensibly' (Hazelhurst 1990: 16). This was ranked above having sex with a girl, learning to swim or drive, being able to talk better to others and getting married. The group coordinator commented: 'It was not realistic to expect most of the young men to survive in the average London pub or disco'

(Hazelhurst 1990: 16). Group visits were made to the cinema, pubs and restaurants.

Hazelhurst's work illustrates the social context of drinking for this group of young men. Visiting a pub is clearly a valued activity but he suggests the young men felt ill-equipped for the social pressure. They had perhaps little experience in going into places containing strangers, lacked confidence in making choices and engaging in appropriate 'small talk' and were not clear about the expectations of 'correct' behaviour and demeanour. Hazelhurst also points out that some pubs can be hazardous places for people who appear vulnerable. Not all pubs have the cosy local neighbourly image portrayed in some television comedies, such as the US comedy *Cheers* or the UK's *Coronation Street*.

In this group work project, attention was given to the challenges faced by the young men with learning disabilities in terms of developing their self-confidence, assertiveness and understanding of their own image as well as acquiring communication skills. The latter included exercises on sustaining conversation, talking to women and managing anger. All these were developed by games and exercises in the supportive environment of the group.

Whilst such projects may use alcohol-associated environments as a typical and valued community activity, they suggest the importance of relating such work to other areas of personal development and learning. The example given above is clearly focused on young men's needs – men who were presumed to be heterosexual, were White and had not lived in long-stay institutions. It is also important, (though not invalidating), to note that they were defined as having moderate learning disabilities and had no physical handicaps or mental illnesses. None the less, such work has particular resonances with early thinking on what normalisation might entail in providing 'normal' or ordinary environments, emphasising that they provide: 'the handicapped adult with the range of conditions and experiences of life that will support his self confidence and feelings of adulthood ... trainees have to acquire self confidence by experiencing themselves as capable of passing over various thresholds of challenge and growth' (Nirje cited in Szivos 1992: 114).

COMMUNITY EDUCATION

Personal diet

It is, of course, important to see alcohol consumption as part of broader health information, though the role of alcohol in general nutrition is often neglected. Rimmer *et al.* (1994) point out that community living must include information about food and diet both as concepts and in practice. Some work is focused on this nutritional axis while other research looks at the product of poor (inadequate or excessive) diet. Bell and Bhate (1992), for example, report that obesity is more prevalent in both male and female populations with learning disabilities than in non-disabled adults. Interestingly their research recommendations are focused on diet as food, rather than noting any possible impact of high-calorie drinks (such as beer), or looking at the patterns of consumption, such as eating food like crisps or nuts with high-calorie drinks.

Alcohol and medication

As with anyone on medication the effect of alcohol in combination with prescribed drugs needs to be discussed with medical personnel. For adults whose care is the responsibility of others this information should be recorded in a care plan which is regularly updated and consulted by all staff and others responsible. People with learning disabilities themselves need to know about the side-effects or dangers of drugs and alcohol. For example Mono Amine Oxidase Inhibitors such as Tranlycypromine or Trifluopolazine are anti-depressant drugs which interfere with the way the body uses Tyramine. A very useful nutritional guide (Brake Brothers 1994) points out that red wine and real ale (amongst other foodstuffs) contain Tyramine and so should be avoided by people using MAOI drugs since they can cause a dangerous rise in blood pressure. Pharmacists should be able to give clear assistance to formal and informal carers about drug reactions and side-effects. They may however need to be alerted to the fact that the person concerned has a degree of choice about diet and that this may include alcohol.

Foetal Alcohol Syndrome (FAS)

While community care services are generally reactive to people's health and social care needs, the issue of public education and prevention of disabilities or ill-health is a more common thread in work with people with addictions. One subject that may need to be recognised by both services is Foetal Alcohol Syndrome (FAS) – a range of symptoms including physical impairment, behavioural problems and intellectual impairment that has been linked to maternal consumption of alcohol.

As McNeil and Litt (1992) report, FAS was only described in 1968 and definitively named in 1973. However, concern over the hereditary nature of learning disabilities has a long history, dating back to the eugenics movement, where 'drunkenness' among women in particular was a sign of moral (and thus racial) degeneracy. Little has changed in this respect as the 'moral panic' over FAS, especially in the US, singles out drinking mothers as culpable and irresponsible.

For workers in community care the debate over FAS and whether control should be exercised over pregnant women and their alcohol consumption is somewhat removed from day-to-day service delivery. However they should be foremost in arguments about the values and prejudices that often arise in such debates. Blaming parents (especially mothers) for the disabilities of their children is no way to run a sensitive and appropriate service.

ALCOHOL PROBLEMS: DEVELOPING A RESPONSE

In this chapter we have described how the cultural context of consuming alcohol has begun to take on positive values. It is ordinary and appropriate for many adults to drink alcohol, though care needs to be taken over issues of gender, religion or cultural preferences that provide other norms of behaviour. However alcohol is not simply a social preference – such as a choice between juice or lemonade. Its content and effects (although often partially socially determined) in many ways loosen inhibitions, 'permit' adults to behave in ways which would otherwise be unacceptable or to undo certain social formalities of behaviour.

This presents a challenge to those whose work essentially involves the teaching and sustained reinforcement of behaviour that *is* socially acceptable and valued. Staff are also aware that for people with learning disabilities, the public gaze plays a very real part in determining attitudes and prejudices.

What then are staff to do when the very activity that is valued in terms of social integration, choice and individuality, leads to behaviour that is disinhibited and perhaps offensive? The first response is to go back to first principles of normalisation to see if such behaviour is being judged on a more harsh scale than it would be for other adults in similar circumstances. The second is to see if there are ways of distinguishing consequences which may have very serious repercussions (the drug/alcohol mix may be fatal), from other unpleasant results (the person may be sick or have a hangover). Third, there is the question of the wider context which may take time but could allow a key worker or care manager to explore why excessive alcohol consumption is playing a major part in the life of someone receiving community care services, if indeed this is the case.

As with many recipients of community care, public and family concerns may be a factor to consider though not necessarily to elevate to primary importance. Parents or neighbours may alert staff to what they consider to be excessive alcohol consumption and inappropriate consequences. Good staff practice will try to ensure their concerns are not dismissed and relationships soured.

Problem drinking

An element of parental disapproval about this aspect of community presence is illustrated by people with learning disabilities in Flynn's research on the lives of eighty-eight people living independently in north-west England in the 1980s. One is reported as being angered by her father:

> 'If me Dad see me in the pub he says, "what the bloody hell are you doing here?" and he sends me out. He doesn't like me going in pubs. Now look at me, I'm twenty-seven and they still treat me like a two-year old. I can't make it out at all.'
>
> (Flynn 1989: 19)

Such a perceptive view reflects the concept outlined by Kurtz (1977) that to be the 'eternal child' is a label often ascribed to people with learning disabilities. In the context of the pub – a

traditionally adult-only environment – the example above illustrates the tension between age as viewed chronologically and
subjectively by the speaker, and her father, who appears both to
deny the adult status of his child and to insist upon a parental
authority out of step in adult relations.

However most people in Flynn's (1989) study, despite their
separation from family life by hospital or hostel residence, did
have regular contact with relatives. Shared activities did include
'going drinking' as well as sharing meals, shopping and going
on outings. In essence, relationships were of similar type to non-
institutionalised individuals.

Some adults with learning disabilities do develop drinking
problems. This is largely unrecorded though we might predict
that as hospitals close and more adults survive, the number may
increase to be more in line with other population groups. One
discussion of a multi-disciplinary Alcohol Education Service in
Dundee describes a four-month treatment programme for adults
with learning disabilities (Lindsay *et al.* 1991). This programme
uses a fairly standard assessment procedure covering reasons for
drinking, drinking situations, alternatives to drinking, knowledge
of alcohol, a drinking diary and a visit to a local pub to see how
the person drinks in real life.

Lindsay *et al.* argue that problems over motivation to reduce
drinking are compounded for people with learning disabilities.
Their treatment programme focuses on giving information and
facilitating changes in behaviour. This latter consists of role-
play or problem-solving sessions (resisting social pressure to
drink), general relaxation and diversionary activities and practice
in pubs. Here clients: 'gain experience of pacing their drinking,
playing pub games and asking for different low alcohol drinks'
(ibid.: 98).

In one of the case examples given, Mr A responded well to the
programme and reduced his alcohol consumption, through
changing his choice of beer. His attendance at the programme
was beneficial in his contact with the police. The researchers
suggest that he was influenced and thus motivated by 'graphic
descriptions of damage that can occur through alcohol and
emphasis on the link between psychological symptoms and alcohol
intake' (ibid.: 99). Although drunk 'now and then', he was
reported as being successfully treated. However in the example
of Mr G, the treatment programme did not seem to have any

sustained affect and Mr G was reported as suffering ill-health, social exclusion and family breakdown as a result of his excessive drinking.

This programme is unusual in that it offers an alcohol-education service to people with learning disabilities, and works with groups in a sustained, long-term relationship. It raises questions about whether alcohol services are ready to respond to people with learning disabilities in terms of knowing their existing community care networks and linking in with the wide variety of services. It also suggests that there are many issues, regardless of disabilities, that need to be considered – such as whether similar group approaches would be appropriate for women or for people who drink in more solitary settings.

Another intervention strategy is outlined by McMurran and Lismore (1993) who used video-tapes as part of specific techniques for reducing drinking. They video-recorded a (role-playing) woman who described her drinking problems and asked two patients at a secure hospital who had learning difficulties to offer concrete advice to the woman. The researchers suggest that the opportunity to give advice generated and reinforced ideas about self-control and alternative activities.

Staff policies in community care

In this final substantive section it is appropriate to consider community care staff's responsibilities and the way these are operationalised by their employers. In some agencies, typically those with a health background or medical aspirations, it is custom and practice that it is unprofessional for staff to drink on duty. For some it is a disciplinary matter. Arguments in favour of this stance centre around the need for staff to behave in a controlled and careful manner that is beyond public reproach. It is in line with practices that remind staff of their liability if something goes wrong and for the need for them to be able to act promptly in emergencies or crises. It is also given as guidance that may protect other staff or service users from harassment or abuse.

At the other extreme are those institutions (of whatever size) where there is a general culture of drinking. Staff and service users are not divided by professional rules but staff may appropriately share the normal pattern of life with service users, acting as friends or companions rather than custodians. Celebrations are jointly undertaken and there is little divide between professional and user. One of these two stereotypes probably resonates with people who have worked in service for people with learning disabilities. The increase in the range of service providers gives opportunities for services to develop on more individual paths, though the role of potential scandal needs to be noted. A serious accident, in which alcohol played a part, might well promote inspectorial concern about safety in this area. Organisations may be questioned about staff behaviour and may find it useful to develop agreed policies about alcohol consumption at work rather than leaving it to an individual manager's preferences.

Community care organisations may also wish to develop policies about home-care services rather than leaving it to individual staff as to whether they shop for alcohol if requested by the client, or assist clients in drinking alcohol if requested. As with all matters of possible risk, both the benefits and hazards should be identified and weighted. Good practice here, as in many areas, notes the importance of discussing matters of concern with others, writing decisions down and monitoring the situation.

CONCLUSION

This chapter has pointed to the symbolic significance of alcohol for people with learning disabilities. In some senses, access to the pub has been seen as a mark of 'normalisation' typically since it is seen to be an ordinary and valued activity. But as we have seen this is not necessarily always or purely positive and people with learning disabilities have just as wide a range of preferences as anyone else. It is likely that as alcohol consumption rises among this group there will be increasing problems as well as benefits. Community care services for people with learning disabilities need to develop links with alcohol services so that such problems are dealt with by ordinary services, that support people with learning disabilities rather than react punitively or stigmatisingly.

REFERENCES

Allen, P. and Scales, K. (1990) 'Promoting residents' rights' in T. Booth (ed.) *Better Lives: Changing Services for People with Learning Difficulties*, Sheffield: Social Services Monographs, University of Sheffield.

Alaszewski, A. and Manthorpe, J. (1991) 'Measuring and managing risk in social welfare', *British Journal of Social Work*, 21: 277–90.

Atkinson, D. (1994) 'I got put away': group-based reminiscence with people with learning difficulties', in J. Bornat (ed.) *Reminiscence Reviewed*, Buckingham: Open University Press.

Bano, A., Crosskill, D., Patel, R., Rashman, L. and Shah, R. (1993) *Improving Practice with People with Learning Disabilities*, London: Central Council for Education and Training in Social Work (CCETSW).

Bell, A. and Bhate, M. (1992) 'Prevalence of overweight and obesity in Down's Syndrome and other mentally handicapped adults living in the community', *Journal of Intellectual Disability Research*, 36: 359–64.

Booth, T. and Booth, W. (1994) *Parenting Under Pressure: Mothers and Fathers with Learning Difficulties*, Buckingham: Open University Press.

Brake Brothers/Home Farm Trust (1994) *Nutritional Guidelines for People with Learning Disabilities*, Ashford, Kent: Brake Brothers.

Brown, H. and Smith, H. (1992) 'Assertion, not assimilation: a feminist perspective on the normalisation principle', in H. Brown and H. Smith (eds) *Normalisation: A Reader for the Nineties*, London: Routledge.

Cahill, M. (1994) *The New Social Policy*, Oxford: Blackwell.

Chappell, A. (1994) 'A question of friendship: community care and the relationship of people with learning difficulties', *Disability and Society*, 9 (4): 419–34.

Craft, M. and Berry, I. (1985) 'The role of the professional in aggression and strategies of coping', in M. Craft., J. Bicknell. and S. Hollins. (eds) *Mental Handicap: A Multi-disciplinary Approach*, London: Ballière Tindall.

Dagnan, D., Howard, B. and Drewett, R. (1994) 'A move from hospital to community-based homes for people with learning disabilities: activities outside the home', *Journal of Intellectual Disability Research*, 38: 567–76.

Emerson, E. (1992) 'Normalisation,' in H. Brown and H. Smith (eds) *Normalisation: A Reader for the Nineties*, London: Routledge.

Flynn, M. (1989) 'The social environment', in A. Brechin and J. Walmsley (eds) *Making Connections*, London: Hodder & Stoughton.

Gilbert, T. (1995) 'Empowerment: issues, tensions and conflicts', in M. Todd and T. Gilbert (eds) *Learning Disabilities – Practice Issues in Health Settings*, London: Routledge.

Hazelhurst, M. (1990) 'Joining the grown-ups', *Community Care*, 15 February: 15–17.

Jahoda, A., Markova, I. and Cattermole, M. (1985) 'Stigma and the self-concept of people with a mild mental handicap', in A. Brechin, and J. Walmsley (eds) *Making Connections*, London: Hodder and Stoughton.

Kurtz, R. (1977) *Social Aspects of Mental Retardation*, Lexington: Lexington Books.

Lindsay, W., Allen, R., Walker, R., Lawrenson, H. and Smith, A. (1991) 'An alcohol education service for people with learning difficulties', *Mental Handicap*, 19, September: 96–100.

McCormack, M. (1979) *Away from Home: the Mentally Handicapped in Residential Care*, London: Constable.

McMurran, M. and Lismore, K. (1993) 'Using video tapes in Alcohol Interventions for people with learning disabilities', *Mental Handicap*, 21: 29–31.

McNeil, M. and Litt, J. (1992) 'More medicalizing of mothers: Foetal Alcohol Syndrome in the USA and related developments', in S. Scott, G. Williams, S. Platt and H. Thomas (eds) *Private Risks and Public Dangers*, Aldershot: Avebury.

Reid, A. (1985) 'Psychiatry and Mental Handicap', in M. Craft, J. Bicknell and S. Hollins (eds) *Mental Handicap: A Multi-disciplinary Approach*, London: Ballière Tindall.

Richardson, A. and Ritchie, J. (1989) *Developing Friendships*, London: Policy Studies Institute.

Richardson, S., Koller, H. and Katz, M. (1994) 'Leisure activities of young adults not receiving mental handicap services who were in a special school for mental handicap as children', *Journal of Intellectual Disability Research*, 38: 163–75.

Rimmer, J., Braddock, D. and Fujiura, G. (1994) 'Cardiovascular risk factors in adults with mental retardation', *American Journal on Mental Retardation*, 98 (4): 515–18.

Szivos, S. (1992) 'The limits to integration', in H. Brown and H. Smith (eds) *Normalisation: A Reader for the Nineties*, London: Routledge.

Shearer, A. (1986) *Building Community with People with Mental Handicaps, their Families and Friends*, London: King's Fund.

Tyne, A. (1992) 'Normalisation: from theory to practice', in H. Brown and H. Smith (eds) *Normalisation: A Reader for the Nineties*, London: Routledge.

Wolf, R. (1990) 'Testimony on behalf of the National Committee for the Prevention of Elder Abuse before the US House Select Committee on Ageing', *Journal of Elder Abuse and Neglect*, 2 (1/2) 137–50.

Wright, K., Haycox, A. and Leedham, I. (1994) *Evaluating Community Care: Services for People with Learning Difficulties*, Buckingham: Open University Press.

Chapter 5

Drinking and homelessness in the UK

Larry Harrison and Hugo Luck

INTRODUCTION

There was a pronounced rise in homelessness in both Britain and the United States throughout the 1970s and 1980s. In the US, this prompted extensive research into the health care needs and increased prevalence of alcohol, drug and mental health problems amongst an increasingly marginalised group; (Ropers and Boyers 1987; Wright and Weber 1987; Breakey *et al.* 1989). US federal government agencies like the National Institute for the Study of Alcohol Abuse and Alcoholism provided substantial funding during the 1980s for demonstration projects designed to improve services for homeless problem drinkers (Argeriou and McCarty 1990).

There has been little to compare to this sustained and comprehensive research effort in the UK, although in the late 1960s Edwards *et al.* (1966, 1968) had highlighted the severe health risks faced by homeless problem drinkers, while Archard's (1979) participant observation study *Vagrancy, Alcoholism and Social Control* offered important insights into the world of the 'bottle gang' or 'drinking school'. These early studies reinforced the contemporary policy concern with habitual drunken offenders (Home Office 1971; DHSS and the Welsh Office 1978) and lent support to a broadly based, though ultimately less than successful, campaign to remove problem drinkers from the penal system (Cook 1975; Out of Court 1982).

By the 1980s however, attention had shifted from alcohol dependence to a wider focus on a range of alcohol-related problems, from drink-driving to soccer violence. There were increasing challenges to stereotypical representations of problem drinkers and to what many felt was an unhelpful preoccupation with the homeless Skid Row 'alcoholic'. The British Government's discussion document *Drinking Sensibly* argued for early identification and treatment, emphasising the fact that the majority of people with drinking problems were in paid employment (DHSS 1981: 60). Concentrating on people who were at a relatively early stage in their drinking career was likely to be more cost-effective than targetting those whose problems had become entrenched.

At the same time, Home Office interest in developing institutional alternatives to prison, like the 'wet shelter', gave way to an emphasis on the extensive use of police cautioning schemes which, it was argued, had been shown to be a more cost-effective way of dealing with drunken offenders (Alcohol Concern 1987). By the late 1980s, the homeless problem drinker had almost disappeared from the UK research agenda; yet paradoxically, down-and-out drinkers had become ever more visible to the general public, due to a rise in street homelessness, together with the loss of some traditional sources of shelter and support and the appearance of large numbers of people sleeping rough in Central London sites like Lincolns Inn Fields. The rise in health and social problems resulting from homelessness was also apparent to clinicians and those providing hostel accommodation, who were struggling to cope with an increasing burden on hard pressed services.

This chapter focuses on the particular problems faced by street drinkers. First, the extent of homelessness and of street drinking are recorded, and the particular health problems faced by homeless people examined. Then the nature and meaning of the links between homelessness and alcohol-related problems are considered, before some implications for service delivery are explored.

THE EXTENT OF HOMELESSNESS

Attempts to estimate the extent of homelessness have been hindered by a lack of agreement over its definition. Narrow definitions of homelessness are concerned with 'rooflessness', which applies to those who lack the most basic shelter. Broader definitions include the residents of institutions who have nowhere else to live: those staying in hostels and bed and breakfast accommodation, and those obliged to live in overcrowded or substandard housing (Greve and Currie 1990). From this point of view, homelessness is best understood as a 'continuum of housing inadequacy and insecurity' (Baumohl 1992).

As with other key concepts in social policy, like poverty, governments favour constricted definitions which minimise official responsibility (Townsend 1979). Thus, local authorities in the UK usually restrict statistics on homelessness to their legal requirement to find housing for those defined as being in 'priority need' under section 3 of the 1985 Housing Act – mainly mothers with dependent children, although there is considerable variation in the way in which different authorities interpret the law (Evans and Duncan 1988).

The numbers of households accepted as being in priority need by local authorities in Great Britain more than doubled in the 1980s: from 75,841 in 1980 to 169,526 in 1990 (Platt 1993). This excludes the 'hidden homeless': those sleeping rough, in night shelters, hostels, prison, squats, staying with family or friends, and in temporary bed and breakfast accommodation.

Although the extent of 'hidden homelessness' is difficult to assess because of the practical difficulties involved in studying a transient population, the 1991 census counted 2,703 sleeping rough on the nights of 21 and 22 April: 1,275 in central London and a further 1,428 in the rest of England and Wales (OPCS 1991).

Many believe this to be a considerable underestimate. Voluntary organisations like Shelter estimated that about 8,000 people were sleeping on the streets of Britain at this time, most of them in London (Platt 1993). A further 4–5,000 single people were believed to be living in bed and breakfast hotels; 11–12,000 in hostels; 10–12,000 in short-life housing; 19,000 squatting in unoccupied property, and an additional 74,000 were overcrowded or unwillingly living in other people's homes (Greve and Currie 1990). Single people made up the greater part of those living in temporary or insecure accommodation.

ALCOHOL PROBLEMS AMONG THE HOMELESS

Levels of alcohol consumption are known to be raised significantly among homeless people seeking health care. A primary health care service aimed at the single homeless in East London (Balazs 1993) found 49 per cent of men (N = 2,101) and 15 per cent of women (N = 485) drinking at high-risk levels. Problem rates among women are generally much lower, but UK estimates of the

Table 5.1   Estimates of the prevalence of alcohol-related problems
among single homeless men in Britain

Investigators	Year	Percentage with alcohol problems	Sample size
Edwards *et al.*	1968	25	279
Priest	1971	16	121
Wood	1976	26*	301
Whynes and Giggs	1989	16.5*	1,573

Note: * Alcohol and drug problems

prevalence of current alcohol-related problems among single homeless men range from 16.5 to 25 per cent (see Table 5.1).

Not included in Table 5.1 is one outlying value: the very low prevalence of current substance problems found by Drake *et al.* (1981: 36) in a study of single homelessness conducted for the Department of the Environment. Drake and colleagues found only 3 per cent of 398 men and 1 per cent of 122 women in England reporting alcohol or drug problems, compared to a typical population value of 6 and 4 per cent respectively (Goddard and Ikin 1988).

This may be partly accounted for by the nature of their sample. Drake and colleagues interviewed men and women in a wide variety of locations, including hotels, boarding houses, bedsits and YMCAs, whereas two of the studies cited in Table 5.1 were of the former Camberwell reception centre (Edwards *et al.* 1968; Wood 1976) while the others sampled the transient population found in soup kitchens, night shelters and hostels. In Drake *et al.*'s study, alcohol or drug-related problems were reported by none of the residents in YMCAs, bedsits and small hostels, compared to 7 per cent of men and women staying in night shelters and 38 per cent of those interviewed in day centres or on soup runs (1981: 75). This suggests that institutional constraints account for at least some of the observed difference: many hostels and bed and breakfast hotels do not accept people with drinking problems.

Moreover, the prevalence rate of 3 per cent in Drake *et al.*'s study refers to those volunteering information about alcohol or drug problems in relation to a question about longstanding disability. Separate questions were asked about drug and alcohol consumption, which show that 11 per cent of 398 men and 3 per cent of 120 women were injecting drug users (ibid.: 41). Alcohol consumption is not reported by gender, but over 11 per cent of 511 men and women appear to have been drinking above the male high-risk level of 50 units per week, compared to 6 per cent of men in the general population (Goddard and Ikin 1988).

With this exception, the UK estimates fall within a relatively narrow range compared to those derived from US studies – which vary from to 2 to 86 per cent (Fischer 1989). However a meta-analysis of sixteen US epidemiological studies claimed lower estimates were associated with better methodology (Lehman and Cordray 1993). Weighted estimates were 28 per cent for current alcohol disorders, which is close to the high end of the British range.

HEALTH NEEDS OF HOMELESS DRINKERS

In the US, it has been established that homeless men and women are at exceptionally high risk for health problems, and this risk is increased substantially by heavy drinking (Ritchey *et al.* 1991; Piliavin *et al.* 1994). In a Los Angeles study, 57 per cent of those defined as homeless alcohol abusers reported chronic health problems compared to 43 per cent of homeless non-abusers (Ropers and Boyers 1987). As Wright and colleagues (1987: 24) noted, 'with few exceptions, rates for virtually every disorder are higher among the alcohol-abusing homeless than among the non-abusers'.

It has been established that there is a close relationship between homelessness and excess morbidity and mortality in the UK, but few studies have examined alcohol effects specifically (for a review see Barry *et al.* 1991). Balazs (1993), for example, showed that rates of medical consultations among homeless men and women were significantly raised for mental health problems, and for cardiovascular, musculoskeletal and dermatological diseases (N = 2,200); he undertook no specific investigation of the inter-relationships between ill health, homelessness and alcohol dependence.

Thirty years ago, Edwards and colleagues noted that out of a random sample of fifty-one problem drinking men, drawn from the regular patrons of a soup kitchen, 16 per cent had been diagnosed as having a peptic ulcer, while 8 per cent had been treated for pulmonary tuberculosis; 6 per cent had lost both legs as a result of accidents, and a further 5 per cent had sustained severe fractures. No less than 20 per cent had attempted suicide. Most respondents were subsisting on an extremely poor diet. Only two (4 per cent) had eaten 'anything approaching a substantial meal' during the twenty-four hours before interview (Edwards *et al.* 1966: 251).

The situation may have improved in the intervening years, but recent surveys indicate that almost half of all street drinkers still receive less than one meal a day, the remainder having erratic or poor diets (Wake 1992). Moore (1987) suggests that malnutrition is far more likely to affect homeless heavy drinkers, and is in turn more difficult to treat. Often the problem is not so much food deficiency, but major dietary imbalance (Koegel *et al.* 1990).

Some recent UK evidence on the health of homeless drinkers comes from a survey of the nature and extent of alcohol-related problems among a sample of 198 men and 114 women known to Irish welfare agencies in England (Harrison and Carr-Hill 1992). A substantial difference in drinking patterns was found between Irish people living in owner-occupied or rented housing and those living in hostels, squats and other forms of insecure accommodation. Like several US studies (see, e.g. Welte and Barnes 1992), Harrison and Carr-Hill found the rate of high-risk drinking for men in transient housing was far higher (29 per cent) than for owner-occupiers (14 per cent). Levels of alcohol dependence were particularly high amongst homeless men: 56 per cent of the sixty-six men in insecure housing and 53 per cent of the sixty men in hostels were identified as alcohol dependent by the Brief Michigan Alcoholism Screening Test (Harrison and Carr-Hill 1992: 39). As in other studies, women in the sample were just as likely to suffer from anxiety and depression as men, but were less likely to drink heavily: only 3.5 per cent of women had current drinking problems (N = 115).

As might be expected, men who were alcohol dependent were significantly more likely than other homeless men to report disorders associated with excessive alcohol consumption, such as chronic liver disease ($\chi^2 = 7.71$ p $\leq$ 0.05), anaemia ($\chi^2 = 5.39$ p $\leq$ 0.05) and hypertension ($\chi^2 = 5.03$ p $\leq$ 0.05). Ulcers and arthritis were also more common among dependent drinkers, but the differences were not statistically significant.

High levels of emotional distress were evident among homeless Irish men and women. While the rate of self-reported depression seemed to decline with age for men, women appeared to suffer another peak of emotional distress when they were over 65 years. Prolonged periods of heavy drinking can result in severe depression and there is a very high suicide rate associated with alcohol dependence (Royal College of Psychiatrists 1986: 75). There was a strong positive correlation between depression and alcohol dependence among men ($\chi^2 = 11.31$ p $\leq$ 0.01).

There appeared to be high levels of heart disease overall. Among 238 people responding to questions on health, fourteen cases of heart disease were recorded – equivalent to a rate of 59 per 1,000 population. Although no precise diagnostic categories were available this appears to be an exceptionally high rate, judged by general practitioner consultation rates for all heart disease of 16.3 per 1,000 population (Royal College of General Practitioners *et al.* 1982). Survey respondents reported a rate three and a half times greater than this.

This may reflect the socioeconomic gradient in heart disease. In 1982 the Standardised Mortality Ratio for coronary heart disease among men aged 20–64 in Great Britain was 70 in social class I, compared to 112 in social class IV and 144 in social class V (OPCS 1986). There have been several specific studies of the reasons for these differences in coronary heart disease mortality and much of the variation can be accounted for by social class differences in the prevalence of smoking and of high blood pressure (Poocock *et al.* 1987; Davey Smith *et al.* 1990). Smoking was much more common among the homeless in Harrison and Carr-Hill's study than among the general population, while those who were alcohol dependent were significantly more likely to report hypertension.

In Struening and Padgett's (1990) investigation of health status among 1,152 homeless men and women in New York City, there were increasing levels of hypertension, heart and circulatory problems as the severity of alcohol and drug problems increased. There is some indication that this may have been the case in Harrison and Carr-Hill's study:

> Those who described themselves as drinking heavily ('daily or frequent heavy drinking sessions') or problematically ('have sought help') were much more likely to have suffered heart problems in the previous 12 months. Fifteen per cent of current heavy and problem drinkers reported heart trouble, compared

to 4.5 per cent of the others. This is probably because heavy drinkers are also much more likely to be smokers, and smoking is a major cause of coronary heart disease.

(Harrison and Carr-Hill 1992: 43)

Even among smokers in their study, however, heavy drinking seemed to be an additional risk factor for heart disease (17 per cent of heavy drinkers compared to 4 per cent of moderate drinkers).

Reanalysis of the survey data shows a strong positive correlation between alcohol dependence and frequent ill health amongst the 115 homeless men. Of the sixty-three homeless men who were dependent on alcohol, 57 per cent had suffered four or more illnesses in the past 12 months, compared to 10 per cent of the fifty-two men who were not dependent ($\chi^2 = 26.01$, $p \leq 0.001$). Alcohol dependence is known to lower resistance to infection and to damage the immune system, and this is likely to show up in vulnerability to a wide range of diseases, including some that are not generally associated with alcohol consumption. It is notable in this connection that in a survey of fifty London street drinkers conducted in the early 1990s, 44 per cent reported a current illness, although only 22 per cent were receiving medical treatment (Wake 1992). Dependent drinking appears to be an additive risk factor amongst the homeless for a variety of diseases.

PERSPECTIVES ON STREET DRINKING

There is general agreement that the demographic characteristics of the homeless population have changed over the last thirty years, with the increasing incidence of homelessness. The 'new homeless' are younger and more heterogeneous than the old Skid Row populations. There is a higher proportion of unmarried and single parent women, adolescents and ethnic minorities (National Institute on Alcohol Abuse and Alcoholism 1989; Greve and Currie 1990). Beyond this assertion of heterogeneity however, there is little agreement on the nature of the problem, and on the most effective and accessible forms of intervention for this new generation of homeless people. In this section we consider the various theoretical perspectives advanced to explain the link between alcohol dependence and homelessness, before outlining some recent developments in service delivery.

Individual level perspectives

In North America some of the earliest sociological studies of people with alcohol-related problems focused on Skid Row – the derelict inner-city areas where single homeless people found cheap accommodation, food and mutual support (Solenberger 1911; Anderson 1923). Much of this literature argued that both problem drinking and homelessness were the result of disaffiliation, the lack of social ties (Bahr 1969). People drifted into Skid Row life because they were not linked into the network of affiliative bonds that provided support and stability for settled persons.

Others saw both disaffiliation and alcohol dependence as being symptoms of an underlying personality disorder. In one of the earliest English studies of a Skid Row population, Edwards and colleagues (1966) found that 58 per cent of their sample of fifty-one men were deprived of a continuing relationship with one or both parents for a period of three or more years before the age of 13. The authors concluded that the lack of social ties observed within this group was not caused in the first instance by heavy drinking but by personality disorder, related to early childhood experience. This vulnerability was combined with an unobstructed drift towards Skid Row, that was partly structured by social class.

Only 6 per cent of Edwards *et al.*'s (1966) sample had been in touch with their families within the past year. In a random sample of 528 homeless people in Baltimore, Breakey *et al.* (1989) also found that problem drinkers were more likely to have severed relations with their family, but not to the same degree as people with severe mental disorders.

Disaffiliation is not a universal finding, however. Bahr (1973) noted that some Skid Row drinkers saw their families relatively frequently: 38 per cent of a sample of 711 men sleeping rough had been in touch with relatives during the past year. Anderson (1987) found that most of the twenty Skid Row women she studied maintained regular contact with their children and friends, despite numerous separations. And a survey of fifty street drinkers conducted for the Arlington Housing Association in London found that many had strong links with the local community and continued to be in regular contact with, and receive support from, family and friends (Wake 1992).

It is possible that some of this variation can be explained by local demographic differences in the populations studied, and by differing criteria for measuring social contact. On this evidence, however, it is by no means clear whether disaffiliation precedes alcohol misuse and homelessness, is a consequence of one or both conditions, or whether the association is spurious.

The homeless problem drinkers in Breakey *et al.*'s (1989) sample were more likely to have a family history of alcohol problems, and showed indications of a more stable background before eventually becoming homeless. Breakey and colleagues believed this lent support to the hypothesis that homelessness was related to a downward drift towards problem drinking, rather than the result of life-long disaffiliation.

Those who favour biological over environmental explanations for alcohol dependence reject the disaffiliation hypothesis with its emphasis on the role of social networks in maintaining people in health. Instead, they regard Skid Row life as one of the consequences of a long-term deterioration in social functioning brought about by severe alcohol dependence. Some evidence seems to support this view. Welte and Barnes (1992) used a covariance structural model to analyse data on homeless people's antecedents, in a random sample of 412 homeless adults. Although alcohol misuse appeared to be a pathway to homelessness, the reverse hypothesis was not supported: homelessness did not seem to precipitate heavy drinking. For a minority, Welte and Barnes argued, drinking had been a contributory cause of their homelessness, but they found no evidence that homelessness led to problem drinking.

Winkleby *et al.* reached different conclusions based on a survey of 1,437 homeless adults in northern California (Winkleby *et al* 1992; Winkleby and White 1992). Prevalences of alcohol abuse, illicit drug use, and psychiatric hospitalisation were 15 to 33 per cent lower when adults first became homeless than following a period of homelessness. Those who reported no impairments when they first became homeless (45 per cent) were likely to develop substance problems and psychiatric disorders over time. Those who had been homeless for over five years reported high rates of alcohol misuse. While some had pre-existing problems, many appear to have become progressively more vulnerable the longer they had lived on the streets.

Wright *et al.* (1987) proposed that homelessness and alcohol dependence combined to generate a unique set of problems. Utilising data from the US Health Care for the Homeless programme, which surveyed over 30,000 people from sixteen different American cities, they found both social and health correlates between homelessness and problem drinking, supporting the hypothesis that homeless people often drink to cope with a traumatic situation. The loss of a home is an extremely stressful life event, and homelessness can be traumatic – the conditions of street and institutional life are stressful, and many become homeless after suffering physical or sexual abuse (Goodman *et al.* 1991: 1219). There is some evidence that homelessness can exacerbate feelings of distrust and social isolation, while the loss of control over key aspects of daily life can reinforce learned helplessness. Thus homelessness can be an additive risk factor for a range of emotional and somatic disorders.

Risk and social structure

New developments in the study of complex social conditions like homelessness and street drinking are likely to be based on the concept of risk rather than of causality. The search for causal explanations has been largely unfruitful, and has been characterised by an exclusive focus on either societal or, more usually, individual factors. The roots of this selective view go back to some of the earliest sociological studies, in which homelessness was divorced from any consideration of social structural factors and identified with Skid Row, which was itself redefined as 'not so much a place as a human condition' (Bahr 1973: 33). A Skid Row neighbourhood was not a concrete historical location, spawned out of inner-city poverty and decay, but an 'isolated and deviant sub-cultural community' (ibid.). Homelessness was defined as 'a condition of detachment from society characterised by the absence or attenuation of the affiliative bonds that link settled persons to a network of interconnected social structures' (ibid.).

The objective condition of homelessness – a social phenomenon that is structured by the employment and housing markets, and by policies adopted towards public housing, poverty, income maintenance and tax relief – became reinterpreted as personal pathology – a 'state of mind', a consequence of the lifestyle and inherent failings of the individual. The homeless person was identified with the hobo, the bum, or the 'rolling stone', part of a deviant minority who could not cope with a normal life style and was unable to accept the ties of human love and friendship.

At an individual level, life history often appears to offer a sufficient explanation for the slow decline into Skid Row life, but at
a collective level it fails to explain why groups who share characteristics like poverty or housing status should be so vulnerable
to tobacco, alcohol and drug-related problems (Cahalan and
Room 1974; Pearson 1987; Harrison and Carr-Hill 1992; Graham
1993; Marsh and McKay 1994).

It is not generally accepted in the UK that there is an association between poverty and high levels of alcohol-related problems,
partly because previous epidemiological evidence has been
ambiguous (Moss and Beresford-Davies 1967; Edwards *et al* 1972a,
1972b), and also because cross-sectional surveys indicate that
average alcohol consumption declines with gross weekly household income (OPCS 1990: 125). The poorest groups are more
likely to abstain, and to drink lightly. As a measure of socioeconomic status, however, household income is known to be affected
by a number of artefacts such as multiple incomes within the
household, regional and industrial differences in wage rates, and
age and gender-related differences in earnings. US surveys which
have adopted more sophisticated measures of socioeconomic
status show that while the proportion of heavy drinkers is similar
in all social classes, alcohol-related *problems* are concentrated
amongst the poorest groups (Cahalan *et al.* 1969). There appears
to be a J-shaped, rather than a linear relationship; it is only the
very poorest groups which show levels of problems substantially
different from others, but the differences between these groups
and the rest are twice as great as between other groups (Cahalan
and Room 1974: 89).

Some contend that these inequalities are the result of social
selection: those who develop drinking problems are unable to
maintain their position in society, it is argued, and drift down the
social scale. While there is some evidence in support of the social
selection hypothesis in relation to long-standing and severe
mental disorders, it is far from conclusive (Brown and Harris
1978; Cochrane 1983), and it is hard to see how selection
could explain similar inequalities that have been observed in the
prevalence of all cause morbidity and mortality (Cochrane and
Stopes-Roe 1980; Townsend and Davidson 1982). Moreover,
although many are receptive to the selection hypothesis where
psychoactive substances like alcohol or heroin are concerned – it
seems quite plausible that severe dependence could be associated

with downward social mobility – it is hard to see how this applies to cigarette smoking, which has the most marked class gradient of all (Marsh and McKay 1994).

It seems more likely that social structural factors like inadequate housing, low income, or unemployment, are major risk factors for a range of physical and psychiatric disorders, in that they expose the poor to continual stress, while limiting access to the material, psychological and social resources required for coping with adversity (Cochrane 1983).

Poverty and homelessness also make people more vulnerable to the harm associated with heavy drinking. In recent years the emphasis within public health on reducing levels of *per capita* alcohol consumption has diverted attention away from variations in vulnerability (Shaw 1979). It is noteable in this regard that it is more common for heavy alcohol consumption to be associated with minimal or no apparent harm in higher socioeconomic groups (Cahalan and Room 1974). This may be because such groups are shielded by better diet, housing, health care and by their higher social status, which makes personal problems easier to manage or less visible. As Harrison and Carr-Hill observed in relation to the Irish community, 'the disadvantaged are more likely to suffer alcohol-related problems, even when drinking at the same levels as more privileged groups, because they lack the material resources, and often the social supports, available to others' (1992: 47).

This is not to argue that drinking problems are structurally determined; rather, it suggests that it is necessary to employ multiple levels of analysis in order to appreciate the interplay between structural factors and individual, family and peer group vulnerabilities and resources (Shinn and Weitzman 1990; Toro *et al* 1991). There also appears to be an interactive process at work, in which disadvantaged groups run greater risks of developing alcohol-related problems, while problem drinking in turn increases the risk of homelessness among marginalised groups: those with alcohol, drug or behavioural problems are likely to be amongst the first to lose out in the competition for low-cost housing. For this reason, the study of street drinking cannot be divorced from a wider consideration of the role of the employment and housing markets, and of government policies towards income maintenance, health, housing and criminal justice (Rossi 1989).

The rapid escalation of street homelessness in recent years is at least in part a consequence of government policies aimed at restricting public expenditure, protecting house prices and promoting alternatives to State housing provision. In the 1980s, British housing policy aimed to encourage home ownership and to overcome housing shortages through market-based solutions. There were major changes in tenure as the numbers of home-owners with a mortgage increased substantially, while there was a sharp decline in the number of households living in rented accommodation (National Audit Office 1990).

In the early 1990s, however, the UK, like Germany and the US, experienced a 'crisis of affordability', with would-be purchasers unable to afford escalating house prices (Bramley 1994). Economic recession, high interest rates and high unemployment led to unprecedented levels of mortgage arrears and repossessions, and of tenants going into debt as a result of deregulation and higher rent levels. The shortage of affordable housing was exacerbated by the sale of 1.5 million council houses in the 1980s, and by a drastic decline in house building – particularly of council house building, which fell from over 100,000 houses per year in the mid 1970s to under 6,000 per year by the early 1990s (Greve and Currie 1990). Changes to social security legislation meant that single people were no longer entitled to assistance with deposits for rented accommodation, while those under 18 were no longer entitled to social security benefits, and those under 25 received a reduced allowance.

A direct effect of these policy changes was to add to the increasing numbers of homeless throughout the country, thereby contributing to a long-term upward trend in which the number of households accepted as homeless by local authorities have multiplied over ten-fold since the 1960s (Greve and Currie 1990). The escalation in the number of families meeting the statutory definition of homelessness has also increased pressure on the single homeless, most of whom are not eligible for help under current legislation. As in the US, 'while millions scrape by or sleep in the vestibule of the shelter system, doubled up with friends and family, hundreds of thousands of the most marginal ... have drifted into the open and remained there' (Baumohl 1992: 8).

By the late 1980s the highly visible increase in the numbers of street sleepers, many of them encamped in temporary settlements in central locations like Lincolns Inn Fields, attracted media criticism. The government responded with an emergency programme of action, designed to 'put an end to concentrations of people sleeping out in city centres' (Department of the Environment 1990). Ministers made it clear that the government attributed the escalation in the numbers of rough sleepers to a breakdown in traditional family relations, thereby implicitly rejecting the evidence from the Department of the Environment's own research which showed clear links between homelessness and poverty (Thomas and Niner 1989).

Despite the allocation of £15 million in 1990–91, intended to provide 1,000 additional bed spaces, the numbers of people sleeping rough did not appear to diminish (Anderson 1993). Faced with this apparent set back, the British Prime Minister explained the persistence of rough sleeping as personal choice, rather than necessity, and in a subsequent election campaign directed specific criticism against the street homeless for 'aggressive begging' (Bates and Simmons 1994).

The UK policy debate is in danger of becoming polarised, as it has done in the US. For the conservative right in America, homelessness is the result of individual and family failure, and the payment of welfare is regarded as a State subsidy for alcohol and drug consumption (Baumohl 1992). Liberals, on the other hand, have located street homelessness in the broader context of poverty and inequality, but have been reluctant to acknowledge high rates of psychopathology and harmful behaviour among the homeless. Such distortions are unhelpful, because they inhibit the development of effective services and policies.

SERVICES FOR STREET DRINKERS

The preceding section shows how radical changes in the housing market in recent years, and an increase in relative poverty, have marginalised the most vulnerable, who are the first to be excluded from low-cost and temporary accommodation. Coupled with the growth in the numbers of the homeless and marginally housed, there has been a lack of specific services for homeless problem drinkers. As a result, this client group frequently moves between tertiary sources of health care, temporary shelter and alcohol treatment services without receiving a comprehensive package of care.

In the US, one response to this problem has been to move beyond crisis intervention and introduce a case (or care) management approach, involving advocacy and the integration of care from a variety of formal and informal networks (see Chapters 3 and 4 for a discussion of the use of case management with people with learning difficulties and older problem drinkers).

Case management for homeless people involves stabilising clients' lives by acting as a 'service broker' in basic support areas such as financial aid and housing (Detrick and Stiepock 1992; Cox et al 1993; Homan et al 1993). Rather than attempting to provide an all-inclusive package of care, case management emphasises the aggressive utilisation of community resources and statutory entitlements. This is in accord with the principle of normalisation, in that it avoids institutionalisation and reduces the risk of labelling service users. Several intensive US case management programmes have been evaluated and appear to be a successful way of rehabilitating, or at least maintaining contact with, service users (Perl and Jacobs 1992; Kirby and Braucht 1993). Successful services often operate on the principle of 'progressive independence'; they begin by ameliorating immediate tangible needs and work towards a collaborative relationship that focuses on other issues, such as drinking problems (Sosin et al. 1993).

One example of an outreach approach in the UK is the service established in East London by the Drink Crisis Centre in 1990. This aims to bridge the gap between the street drinking population and existing alcohol services in order to create a more coordinated response (Freimanis 1993: 119). It combines day centre provision with outreach work in order to contact as many potential service users and providers as possible. The project attempts to raise the self-esteem of clients, enabling them to identify and develop appropriate coping strategies (Freimanis 1993: 122). It also works with staff in established services for the homeless in order to promote a greater understanding of the knowledge and skills required for working with problem drinkers. Such an outreach service provides a flexible, pragmatic way of working which offers an effective alternative to, and augmentation of, more static services.

In the past many residential rehabilitation facilities were aimed solely at the treatment of problem drinking. They made little attempt to tackle the issue of homelessness – offering little more than a temporary respite for homeless problem drinkers (Dunne

1990). In recent years more specialist provision for homeless problem drinkers has been developed, much of it designed to support abstinence. In the US, for example, Alcohol-Free Living Centres provide a low-rent, alcohol-free environment for homeless people who are trying to achieve abstinence. Koroloff and Anderson (1989) evaluated the effectiveness of an Alcohol-Free Living Centre in Portland, Oregon. Data were collected on eighty clients whose average length of stay in the living centre was 89 days. Clients who completed the programme were admitted less often to, and spent significantly fewer days in, short-term detoxification. These reductions occurred whether or not the clients successfully completed the treatment plan while living at the centre. By the end of the programme, there were also substantial changes in employment status, income, and perceived employability.

In the UK, there has also been emphasis on abstinence as the primary goal of intervention, and most mainstream accommodation will neither accept homeless people who continue drinking nor continue to provide shelter for those who relapse. While this policy protects a small group of homeless drinkers who are trying to change their circumstances, it condemns others to a precarious existence by making the right to accommodation dependent on the individual's successful functioning.

Alcohol Concern, the UK's national alcohol agency, has argued for a range of different accommodation, both for those who choose to live their lives free of alcohol and for those who are not able to achieve that goal. In 1987 Alcohol Concern outlined four initiatives aimed at helping the homeless problem drinker: the creation of crisis centres, providing overnight accommodation for drunken offenders; increased availability of long-term supported housing, without rigid rules concerning drinking behaviour; good hostel accommodation for problem drinkers; and improved links between the residential and housing sectors (1987).

The experience of other countries indicates that such services should be accessible, not merely in terms of geographic proximity, but through reducing social distance, role expectations, and organisational rules, in order to make the alienation of service users less frequent (Baumohl and Heubner 1991). Some British agencies have attempted to provide such a service and appear to have met with initial success. These projects have recognised that abstinence is not a realistic objective for many service users, and that to pursue this goal to the exclusion of all others is a fruit-less and often costly task. It is important to encourage those who cannot stop drinking to adopt less harmful behaviours and to keep them in contact with those who offer health care or help over drinking. Five projects are described here, two offering long-term accommodation, the third day centre services, and the fourth and fifth a programme of supported housing. All offer a service which attracts, rather than excludes, the homeless problem drinker.

The First Peterloo Heavy Drinkers' Project

The heavy drinkers project of the First Peterloo Housing Association initially consisted of a house which provided accom-modation for eight men in single rooms. It expanded in 1990 to include a further sixteen beds in two- and three-bedroomed terraced houses. The project's aim was to provide long stay care for homeless problem drinkers, especially those who had become dependent upon crude spirits. Each unit provided four distinct features:

1 single rooms were provided for all residents, with some communal facilities;
2 house rules were kept to a minimum;
3 drinking was allowed on the premises;
4 one meal a day was provided by staff to ensure nutritional needs of the residents were met.

(First Peterloo Housing Association 1993)

At the time of writing insufficient time has elapsed for outcome evaluation, and few definite conclusions can be drawn as to success or failure of the project, but an initial report indicated a number of promising outcomes:

1 four residents had stopped drinking altogether and had moved into 'dry' accommodation;
2 a noticeable decline had taken place in the consumption of surgical spirits;
3 several residents had renewed contact with their families, in one instance after a period of twenty-seven years;
4 the number of violent episodes involving residents had decreased;
5 standards of personal health and hygiene had improved;

6   none of the residents had been arrested for alcohol-related
    offences during their time with the project.

                                    (Rossington and Cameron 1993)

The project took a calculated risk in permitting drinking under
controlled conditions within its houses. This harm minimisation
approach allowed residents a considerable amount of independence and ensured that their housing status was not placed in
jeopardy by their drinking behaviour. In response, some residents
seem to have reduced harmful drinking practices.

Aspinden Wood

A similar venture opened in South-East London in 1992 as a result
of collaboration between the Drink Crisis Centre, a non-statutory
alcohol agency, and a housing association (Bennett 1994).
Aspinden Wood is a purpose-built, high-care, eighteen-bed registered care home for street drinkers, which offers long-term
residents both a 'wet' and a 'dry' lounge. Staff provide food,
laundry and medication. After two years of operation there
had been no violent incidents and although the 'wet lounge'
was described as having a 'battered' appearance, the property
remained in good condition overall (Bennett 1994).

The Handel Street Day Centre

Like other large cities in the UK, Nottingham has a sizable homeless population. A study by Whynes and Giggs (1992) reported
that from June 1988 to August 1989 over 2,000 people contacted
relevant agencies in the city of Nottingham requesting shelter or
assistance with housing.

In 1990 the City Council and Nottingham Help the Homeless attempted to address the needs of street drinkers by
opening the Handel Street Day Centre (Williams 1992). The aims
of this project were to provide shelter during the day, with no
pressure to move on elsewhere for homeless problem drinkers,
and to provide hot food and drink and access to primary health
care, while indirectly decreasing the likelihood of offending
behaviour.

The Centre was one of the first to permit drinking on the
premises, with the proviso that the contents of glass bottles were

decanted into plastic containers. Morrish (1993: 45) reports that such precautions, together with an overall attitude of tolerance held by staff, contributed to very low levels of violence. This permissive attitude to drinking did not appear to encourage higher levels of consumption. Many took advantage of the health and other facilities offered, and though little is known yet of the long-term outcomes, it appears that the agency has ameliorated many of the harsher aspects of life for homeless problem drinkers in Nottingham and has drawn attention to the scale of the problem locally.

Supported housing: the DCC and ARP

Supported housing is an alternative which aims to reintegrate street drinkers into the community. The Drink Crisis Centre offers support to a number of flats owned by housing associations. Each resident has an individual care package, with visiting housing support workers providing advice and life skills training. The Alcohol Recovery Project is also developing a programme of 'floating care', in which support is gradually withdrawn as residents become better able to care for themselves (Bennett 1994).

CONCLUSION

The projects described above have shown that it is possible to reduce the level of harm experienced by some of the most vulnerable and chaotic street drinkers, and represent the first building blocks in an evolving pattern of care: from outreach services to crisis centres, 'wet' hostels, sheltered housing and alcohol-free living centres. Ideally it should be possible for service users to move between accommodation units according to their needs, so that those who relapse while staying in 'dry' accommodation do not have to return to the street, but move instead to a unit which is able to work with continuing drinkers. This kind of integrated continuum of care is being developed in some American cities. The continuum of care needs to be underpinned by an active case management approach to help clients obtain welfare benefits, job counselling and employment opportunities. Case managers can also ensure coordination with, as well as offering support and advice to, staff in mainstream housing, health and social services.

Many hostels for the homeless have been placed under great strain since the 1980s, because escalating levels of problem drinking have posed acute management problems for hostel staff (Harrison and Carr-Hill 1992). At the same time, some alcohol treatment services have been less effective than they might have been because they have paid insufficient attention to the housing problems experienced by service users. This is the legacy of past theoretical formulations of both homelessness and alcohol dependence, which have adopted an individual focus and under-emphasised the social context within which such problems arise. Homelessness, in particular, is a condition 'rooted in economic and social relations' (Baumohl and Heubner 1991: 856).

A comprehensive analysis is needed which can explain the interaction between biography, culture, and social structure. This would direct attention to the way in which the operation of the employment and housing markets, and the consequences of government intervention, have generated conditions which foster high levels of street drinking. British housing policy, for example, has neglected the needs of single homeless people – the government resorting to emergency measures only when the problem of rough sleeping became a political embarrassment (Anderson 1993). Even a partial resolution of the problems of street homelessness and street drinking requires more than short-term, emergency initiatives: like other areas of social welfare, it requires preventive action across a broad front, involving policies on housing, health, income support, employment, education and training (see Chapter 10).

If concerted action was taken now to reduce the incidence of homelessness and street drinking, considerable numbers of homeless people would continue to avoid, or be excluded from, essential services because of their drinking behaviour. For the foreseeable future the need for innovative services of the kind described in this chapter is likely to grow. Prevention and treatment are not alternatives.

REFERENCES

Alcohol Concern (1987) *Alcohol Services – The Future*, London: Alcohol Concern.

Anderson, I. (1993) 'Housing policy and street homelessness in Britain', Housing Studies, 8(1): 17–28.

Anderson, N. (1923) *The Hobo: The Sociology of the Homeless Man*, Chicago: University of Chicago Press.

Anderson, S. C. (1987) 'Alcoholic women on skid row', *Social Work*, 32(4): 362–5.

Archard, P. (1979) *Vagrancy, Alcoholism and Social Control*, London: Macmillan.

Argeriou, M. and McCarty, D. (eds) (1990) *Treating Alcoholism and Drug Abuse Among Homeless Men and Women*, New York: Haworth Press.

Bahr, H. M. (1969) 'Lifetime affiliation patterns of early and late onset heavy drinkers on Skid Row', *Quarterly Journal of Alcohol Studies*, 30: 645–56.

Bahr, H. M. (1973) *Skid Row: An Introduction to Disaffiliations*, New York: Oxford University Press.

Balazs, J. (1993) 'Health care for single homelessness people', in K. Fisher and J. Collins (eds) *Homelessness, Health Care and Welfare Provision*, London: Routledge.

Barry, A., Carr-Hill, R. and Glanville, J. (1991) *Homelessness and Health*, Centre for Health Economics Discussion Paper 84, York: University of York.

Bates, S. and Simmons, M. (1994) 'PM attacks "offensive" beggars', *Guardian*, 28 May: 1.

Baumohl, J. (1992) 'Addiction and the American debate about homelessness', *British Journal of Addiction*, 87(1): 7–10.

Baumohl, J. and Heubner, R. (1991) 'Alcohol and other drug problems among homeless: research, practice and future directions', *Housing Policy Debate*, 2: 837–66.

Bennett, M. (1994) 'Street drinkers come in from the cold', *Alcohol Concern Magazine*, 9(4): 12–13, 15.

Bramley, G. (1994) 'An affordability crisis in British housing: dimensions, causes and policy impact', *Housing Studies*, 9(1): 103–24.

Breakey, W. R., Fischer, P. J., Kramer, M., Nestadt, G., Romanoski, A. J., Ross, A., Royall, R. M. and Stine, O. C. (1989) 'Health and mental-health problems of homeless men and women in Baltimore', *Journal of the American Medical Association*, 262(10): 1352–7.

Brown, G. W. and Harris, T. O. (1978) *Social Origins of Depression*, London: Tavistock.

Cahalan, D., Cisin, I. H. and Crossley, H. M. (1969) *American Drinking Practices: A National Study of Drinking Behavior and Attitudes*, New Brunswick, NJ: Rutgers Center for Alcohol Studies.

Cahalan, D. and Room, R. (1974) *Problem Drinking Among American Men*, New Brunswick, NJ: Rutgers University Press.

Cochrane, R. (1983) *The Social Creation of Mental Illness*, Harlow: Longman.

Cochrane, R. and Stopes-Roe, M. (1980) 'Factors effecting the distribution of psychological symptoms in urban areas of England', *Acta Psychiatrica Scandinavica*, 61: 445–60.

Cook, T. (1975) *Vagrant Alcoholics*, London: Routledge & Kegan Paul.

Cox, G. B., Meijer, L., Carr, D. I. and Freng, S. A. (1993) 'Systems alliance and support (SAS): a program of intensive case management for chronic public inebriates: Seattle', *Alcoholism Treatment Quarterly*, 3(4): 125–38.

Davey Smith, G., Shipley, M. and Rose, G. (1990) 'The magnitude and causes of socio-economic differentials in mortality: further evidence from the Whitehall study', *Journal of Epidemiology and Community Health*, 44(4): 256–70.

Department of Health and Social Security (DHSS) (1981) Prevention and Health: *Drinking Sensibly*, London: HMSO.

Department of Health and Social Security and the Welsh Office (1978) *The Pattern and Range of Services for Problem Drinkers: Report of the Advisory Committee on Alcoholism*, London: HMSO.

Department of the Environment (1990) 'Michael Spicer Unveils £15 Million Plan to Tackle Single Homelessness', *Department of the Environment News Release*, London: DoE.

Detrick, A. and Stiepock, V. (1992) 'Treating persons with mental illness, substance abuse, and legal problems: the Rhode Island experience', *New Directions for Mental Health Services*, 56 (Winter): 65–77.

Drake, M., O'Brien, M. and Biebuyck, T. (1981) *Single and Homeless*, London: HMSO.

Dunne, F. J. (1990) 'Alcohol abuse on skid row: in sight out of mind', *Alcohol and Alcoholism*, 25(1): 13–5.

Edwards, G., Chandler, J., Hensman, C. and Peto, J. (1972a) 'Drinking in a London suburb. I, correlates of normal drinking', *Quarterly Journal of Studies on Alcohol*, 6: 69.

Edwards, G., Chandler, J., Hensman, C. and Peto, J. (1972b) 'Drinking in a London suburb. II, correlates of trouble with drinking among men', *Quarterly Journal of Studies on Alcohol*, 6: 94.

Edwards, G., Hawker, A., Williamson, V. and Hensman, C. (1966) 'London's Skid Row', *Lancet*, 1: 249–52.

Edwards, G., Williamson, V., Hawker, A., Hensman, C. and Postyan, S. (1968) 'Census of a reception centre', *British Journal of Psychiatry*, 114: 1031–9.

Evans, A. and Duncan, S. (1988) *Responding to Homelessness: Local Authority Policy and Practice*, London: HMSO.

First Peterloo Housing Association (1993) *The First Peterloo Heavy Drinkers Project*, Manchester: First Peterloo Housing Association.

Fischer, P. J. (1989) 'Estimating the prevalence of alcohol, drug and mental health problems in the contemporary homeless population: a review of the literature', *Contemporary Drug Problems*, 16(3): 333–89.

Freimanis, L. (1993) 'Alcohol and single homelessness: an outreach approach', in K. Fisher and J. Collins (eds) *Homelessness, Health Care and Welfare Provision*, London: Routledge.

Goddard, E. and Ikin, C. (1988) *Drinking in England and Wales in 1987*, London: HMSO.

Goodman, L., Saxe, L. and Harvey, M. (1991) 'Homelessness as a psychological trauma: broadening perspectives', *American Psychologist*, 46(11): 1219–25.

Graham, H. (1993) *When Life's a Drag: Women, Smoking and Disadvantage*, London: HMSO.

Greve, J. and Currie, E. (1990) *Homelessness in Britain*, York: Joseph Rowntree Trust.

Harrison, L. and Carr-Hill, R. (1992) *Alcohol and Disadvantage amongst the Irish in England*, London: Federation of Irish Societies.

Homan, S. M., Flick, L. H., Heaton, T. M., Mayer, J. P. and Klein, M. (1993) 'Reaching beyond crisis management: design and implementation of extended shelter-based services for chemically dependent homeless women and their children', *Alcoholism Treatment Quarterly*, 3(4): 101–12.

Home Office (1971) *Habitual Drunken Offenders: Report of the Working Party*, London: HMSO.

Kirby, M. J. and Braucht, G. N. (1993) 'Intensive case management for homeless people with alcohol and other drug problems: Denver', *Alcoholism Treatment Quarterly*, 3(4): 187–200.

Koegel, P., Burnam, M. and Farr, R. (1990) 'Subsistence adaptation among homeless adults in the inner city of Los Angeles', *Journal of Social Issues*, 46(4): 83–107.

Koroloff, N. M. and Anderson, S. C. (1989) 'Alcohol-Free Living Centers: hope for homeless alcoholics', *Social Work*, 34(6): 497–504.

Lehman, A. F. and Cordray, D. S. (1993) 'Prevalence of alcohol, drug, and mental disorders among the homeless: one more time', *Contemporary Drug Problems*, 20(3): 355–83.

Marsh, A. and McKay, S. (1994) *Poor Smokers*, London: Policy Studies Institute.

Moore, D. T. (1987) 'A class lesson in alcoholic malnutrition: the poor get sicker than the affluent', *Alcohol Health and Research World*, 11(4).

Morrish, P. (1993) *Living in the Shadows: The Accommodation Needs and Preferences of Homeless Heavy Drinkers*, Leeds: Accommodation Forum.

Moss, M. C. and Beresford-Davies, E. (1967) *A Survey of Alcoholism in an English County*, London: Geigy.

National Audit Office (1990) *Homelessness: Report by the Comptroller and Auditor General*, London: HMSO.

National Institute on Alcohol Abuse and Alcoholism (1989) *Homelessness, Alcohol, and Other Drugs*, Rockville, Md: National Institute on Alcohol Abuse and Alcoholism.

Office of Population Censuses and Surveys (OPCS) (1986) *Occupational Mortality, The Registrar General's Decennial Supplement for Great Britain*, Series DS No. 6, London: HMSO.

Office of Population Censuses and Surveys (OPCS) (1990) *General Household Survey 1988*, London: HMSO.

Office of Population Censuses and Surveys (OPCS) (1991) *1991 Census Preliminary Report for England and Wales: Supplementary Monitor on People Sleeping Rough*, London: HMSO.

Out of Court (1982) *Dealing with Drunkenness: a Proposal for Change*, London: FARE.

Pearson, G. (1987) *The New Heroin Users*, London: Blackwell.

Perl, H. I. and Jacobs, M. L. (1992) 'Case management models for homeless persons with alcohol and other drug problems: an overview of the NIAAA research demonstration program', in R. Ashery (ed.) *Progress and Issues in Case Management*, NIDA Research Monograph, Rockville, Md: NIDA.

Piliavin, I., Westerfelt, A., Wong, Y. and Afflerbach, A. (1994) 'Health status and health care utilization among the homeless', *Social Service Review*, 68(2): 236–53.

Platt, S. (1993) 'Without walls', *New Statesman and Society*, 2 April: 5–7.

Poocock, S., Shaper, A., Cook, D., Philips, A. and Walker, M. (1987) 'Social class differences in ischaemic heart disease in British men', *Lancet*, ii: 197–201.

Ritchey, F. J., Lagory, M. and Mullis, J. (1991) 'Gender differences in health risks and physical symptoms among the homeless', *Journal of Health and Social Behavior*, 32(1): 33–48.

Ropers, R. H. and Boyers, R. (1987) 'Homelessness as a health risk', *Alcohol Health and Research World*, 11(3): 38–41, 89.

Rossi, P. (1989) *Down and Out in America: The Origins of Homelessness*, Chicago: University of Chicago Press.

Rossington, J. and Cameron, R. (1993) *No Place Like Home*, London: Alcohol Concern.

Royal College of General Practitioners, OPCS and Department of Health (1982) Morbidity Statistics from General Practice, 1981–82, *Third national study: socio-economic analyses*, London: HMSO.

Royal College of Psychiatrists (1986) *Alcohol: Our Favourite Drug*, London: Tavistock.

Shaw, S. (1979) 'Epidemiology', in M. Grant and P. Gwinner (eds) *Alcoholism in Perspective*, London: Croom Helm.

Shinn, M. and Weitzman, B. (1990) 'Research on homelessness: an introduction', *Journal of Social Issues*, 46(4): 1–11.

Solenberger, A. (1911) *One Thousand Homeless Men*, New York: Russell Sage Foundation.

Sosin, M. R., Schwingen, J. and Yamaguchi, J. (1993) 'Case management and supported housing in Chicago: the interaction of program resources and client characteristics', *Alcoholism Treatment Quarterly*, 3(4): 35–50.

Struening, E. L. and Padgett, D. K. (1990) 'Physical health status, substance use and abuse, and mental disorders among homeless adults', *Journal of Social Issues*, 46(4): 65–81.

Thomas, A. and Niner, P. (1989) *Living in Temporary Accommodation: A Survey of Homeless People*, London: HMSO.

Toro, P., Trickett, E., Wall, D. and Salem, D. (1991) 'Homelessness in the United States: an ecological perspective', *American Psychologist*, 46(11): 1208–18.

Townsend, P. (1979) *Poverty in the United Kingdom: a Survey of Household Resources and Standards of Living*, Harmondsworth: Penguin.

Townsend, P. and Davidson, N. (eds) (1982) *Inequalities in Health: The Black Report*, Harmondsworth: Penguin.

Wake, M., (ed.) (1992) *Homelessness and Street Drinking*, London: Arlington Housing Association.

Welte, J. W. and Barnes, G. M. (1992) 'Drinking among homeless and marginally housed adults in New York State', *Journal of Studies on Alcohol*, 53(4): 303–15.

Whynes, D. K. and Giggs, J. A. (1992) 'The health of the Nottingham homeless', *Public Health*, 106(4): 307–14.

Williams, J. (1992) *The Handel Street Day Centre for Homeless Street Drinkers: The First Year*, Nottingham: Nottingham University Press.

Winkleby, M. A., Rockhill, B., Jatulis, D. and Fortmann, S. P. (1992) 'The medical origins of homelessness', *American Journal of Public Health*, 82(10): 1394–8.

Winkleby, M. A. and White, R. (1992) 'Homeless adults without apparent medical and psychiatric impairment: onset of morbidity over time', *Hospital and Community Psychiatry*, 43(10): 1017–23.

Wood, S. M. (1976) 'Camberwell Reception Centre: a consideration of the need for health and social services of homeless single men', *Journal of Social Policy*, 5(4): 389–99.

Wright, J. D., Knight, J. W., Weber, B. E. and Lam, J. (1987) 'Ailments and alcohol: health status among the drinking homeless', *Alcohol Health and Research World*, 11(3): 22–7.

Wright, J. D. and Weber, E. (1987) *Homelessness and Health*, New York: McGraw-Hill.

Chapter 6

Social influences on treatment outcomes

Roger Marshall

INTRODUCTION

Despite increasing evidence which highlights the 'significant prevalence' of clients with alcohol-related problems in the social
worker's caseload (Abel 1983; Leckie *et al.* 1984; Leckie 1990),
the majority of social workers have confined their professional
involvement to supporting family members who are most affected
by the drinker's behaviour, and to carrying out their statutory
child protection role (Isaacs and Moon 1985). In a survey which
involved a cross-section of social workers, it was reported that:
'responses intended to help the problem drinker counter difficulties with drink usually involved bringing in a third party. Often
this would be the GP' (Isaacs and Moon 1985: 38). Other sources
of help utilised by the social worker – which involved referring
clients to Alcohol Treatment Units or to meetings of Alcoholics
Anonymous (AA) – often provoked hostility from their clients,
many of whom rejected the process of being labelled an 'alcoholic' (Shaw *et al.* 1978).

In addition to a lack of training in addictions which many social
workers pin-point as the reason for their lack of confidence in
responding adequately to clients with alcohol-related problems,
Hebblethwaite (1979) noted that the belief held by many social
workers that alcohol dependence is a medical problem which
requires specialist medical treatment, is combined with the
absence of a legislative framework which would enable social work
to accept responsibility for the organisation and delivery of
services in the alcohol field.

The movement away from a judgemental approach which
punished the problem drinker, towards a conception of alcoholism

as a disease which requires medical attention, initially represented an advance in the societal response to problem drinkers. Although this view is still widely held (Royal College of Psychiatrists 1979: 56) it has been called into question in recent years by those who view alcoholism as an addictive behaviour (Miller *et al.* 1980; Orford 1985). From this perspective, Orford argues that continued adherence to the medical model of alcoholism has retarded our understanding of the commonalities which exist between a variety of addictive behaviours. The emphasis which the medical model places on the primacy of medical intervention – necessitating the attention of medical specialists – has also hampered the development of an effective social work response to the many clients in the community who are unwilling, or due to the scarcity of alcohol treatment are unable, to receive medical treatment for their condition.

For these reasons this chapter will focus on factors which are thought to be responsible for the attainment and maintenance of remission from alcohol-related problems when formal intervention is absent, in the belief that by gaining a better understanding of the factors involved in the spontaneous remission process, social workers will be able to develop a framework of care for problem drinkers in the community.

This chapter is divided into three parts. In part one, literature which presents evidence for the existence and frequency of spontaneous remission will be reviewed. This is followed in part two by a review of the evidence that intensive treatment cannot be shown to be more effective in the attainment of long-term remission from alcohol-related problems than minimal or no treatment. Part three will review the factors which were cited as important to remission in longitudinal studies of treated and untreated problem drinkers, in order to discover what influence a longer time frame has on the reporting of remission factors.

PART ONE

Spontaneous remission from alcohol-related problems

Part one begins by outlining the reasons for the importance of studying spontaneous remission and some of the methodological problems which hamper research in this area. According to Roizen *et al.* (1978), the study of spontaneous remission from alcohol-related problems is important because if no reliable information exists about the frequency rate of spontaneous remission, the effectiveness of treatment regimes cannot be established since there is no base-line against which the effectiveness of treatment can be measured. Roizen *et al.* argue, therefore, that treatment success rates cannot be used as a test of their own conceptual foundations in the absence of greater knowledge about spontaneous remission rates.

Spontaneous remission also touches on two central areas of debate within the field of alcohol studies, the first of which is that by its very existence, spontaneous remission could call into question some of the core assumptions about the natural history of alcoholism made by the adherents of the disease model. This model views alcohol dependence as an irreversible condition defined by the presence of an abnormal craving which, if it is not checked by treatment and a life-long commitment to abstinence, will result in progressive deterioration. The alcoholic is viewed as being genetically different from the non-alcoholic and can therefore never return to a controlled or asymptomatic form of social drinking (Davies and Raistrick 1981; Heather and Robertson 1985). Roizen *et al.* note: 'where alcoholism is regarded as a progressive and irreversible condition, spontaneous remission also indicates the degree to which either the progressive characterisation or the diagnostic criteria for alcoholism require rethinking and revision' (1978: 198).

Second, the experience of untreated alcoholics would act as an important control on the influence of clinical ideology on the question of whether a return to controlled drinking is a feasible goal (ibid.).

Another equally important reason for studying the process of spontaneous remission is that the research undertaken into the success rates of formal treatment for alcohol dependence show many treatments to be either ineffective, unproven or only modestly effective in securing the attainment of long-term remission. Saunders and Allsop cite Mulford's observation that 'none of the dozens of formal treatments for alcoholism appear to be either necessary or sufficient for recovery' (Saunders and Allsop 1986: 205).

Miller and Hester adopted a more cautious approach to the evaluation of treatment effectiveness. When concluding their own extensive review of the literature on alcohol problems they wrote: 'the majority of treatment procedures for problem drinkers

warrant a "Scotch verdict" of unproved at the present time'
(Miller and Hester 1980: 108). In a more recent review of treatment evaluation, Miller and Hester (1986) found empirical
evidence to support the effectiveness of some treatment modalities, which suggests that a more optimistic view should be taken
of the role of intervention. Further evidence to support this
view can be found in several other recent studies, including Holder
et al. (1991) and McCrady (1991).

It is worth noting that those modalities which were most
strongly supported by the evidence in each of these studies
concentrate on psychological and social interventions which can
be provided in non-medical settings within the community. Against
such a background there may be processes at work in the case of
untreated remitters which could be incorporated into treatment
programmes to improve their effectiveness – or at least to increase
our understanding of factors that may be used to augment formal
treatment.

The subject of spontaneous remission from alcohol-related
problems is a controversial one, and its existence and frequency
are contested. Eysenck and Beech have argued that because of
the supposed nature of alcoholism, 'spontaneous remission is
theoretically expected to be almost entirely absent, and clinical
experience certainly suggests that a lack of treatment would almost
always mean an absence of improvement'(1971: 586).

Others have argued that alcohol-related problems principally
afflict the younger members of a population, most of whom will
'mature out' of the problem by the time they have reached their
mid-40s without the aid of treatment. So alcohol dependence is
viewed as a self-limiting disease for the majority of individuals
(Drew 1968), which might even be sub-culturally normal for some
(Room 1977). From this perspective, treatment would only be
required for the small proportion of people who continue to drink
heavily into their forties and beyond. Tuchfeld (1981) observes
that attempts have been made to reconcile these contradictory
perspectives on rates of spontaneous remission by postulating the
existence of an addictive alcoholic type, who is unable to gain
remission independently of treatment, and a non-addictive type,
for whom the processes involved in spontaneous remission will
be sufficient.

An example of the concept of the alcohol addict can be found
in Jellinek's classification of alcoholic types, and particularly in

the *gamma* category of alcoholism which he argued was the most prevalent form of alcoholism in Britain and America. Gamma alcoholism is characterised as a condition in which: 'there is a definite progression from psychological to physical dependence and marked behaviour changes' (Jellinek 1960: 37).

This argument would suggest that treatment would be a necessary factor for remission of only the most severe cases of alcohol dependence, but as Tuchfeld notes: 'increasingly, however, empirical evidence suggests that untreated resolutions occur regardless of diagnostic severity' (Tuchfeld 1981: 627).

Differences between reported rates of spontaneous remission

Widely varying rates of spontaneous remission have been reported in the literature. For example, Kissin *et al.* (1968), in a comparative study of three different treatments, reported that only 4 per cent of the fifty untreated cases of alcoholism which constituted their control group could be counted as showing any improvement in their drinking habits. This figure may be contrasted with the comparatively high rates of spontaneous remission reported in Goodwin *et al.*'s (1971) retrospective study of a prison population of alcoholics, who when interviewed at an 8-year follow up were found to have a 40 per cent remission rate. Three more studies which reported high rates of spontaneous remission are Robson *et al.* (1965), Clancy (1961); and Clancy *et al.* (1965): these reported improvement rates of 37 per cent, 40 per cent and 54 per cent respectively.

The personal characteristics and social factors which have been held to account for these wide variations in the reported improvement outcome among untreated samples of problem drinkers will be reviewed later, although it is noted here that Kreitman (1977: 50) has advised that studies which offer explanations of differences in self-reported drinking behaviour as being attributable entirely to social class must be viewed with 'extreme circumspection'. Although under-reporting of alcohol consumption is common, it is most marked in heavy drinkers, and the middle class are less honest in reporting their alcohol intake than are working-class respondents.

A further important factor which may shed light on the wide variations that exist in reported rates of spontaneous remission is the lack of consensus which exists within the field of alcohol studies over a definition of what constitutes an 'alcoholic' or a 'problem drinker', or what the criteria might be for differentiating between these two labels. In addition to the problems of differences in the time interval chosen for follow-up, and differences in diagnostic criteria between studies (and the sample selection bias which may result from this), a lack of consensus also exists about the criteria which must be adopted in defining a successful drinking outcome.

Roizen *et al.* (1978) carried out their own survey of a general population sample to discover what the effects would be if different diagnostic criteria were used to define alcoholism, and the criteria chosen for scoring successful remission were varied, when applied to the same data. They undertook a two-wave panel study consisting of a lengthy interview at time 1, and a follow-up interview at time 2, four years later. The total sample of untreated problem drinkers equalled 521 in both cases.

At their first interview, 39 per cent of the sample had at least one problem with their drinking. If the criteria for remission were limited to those respondents with severe problems at time 1 who had achieved no problems at time 2, a low remission rate (11 per cent) would have been recorded. However, by successively relaxing the remission criteria to include those subjects with a drop of one or more points in their initial problem score at time 2, the remission rate rose to 71 per cent of the sample. Roizen *et al.* concluded that due to an absence of consensus regarding the criteria which should be applied to distinguish between the 'alcoholics' and 'problem drinkers' in their sample, no natural boundary could exist to differentiate between remission and non-remission from alcohol-related problems and that 'therefore, the notion of remission can be equated with a variety of more or less arbitrary standards falling between abstinence at one extreme and "any improvement" at the other' (1978: 214).

Possible causes of spontaneous remission

This section will begin by reviewing some of the factors which were found to be associated with spontaneous remission from alcohol-related problems in spontaneous remitters who were identified in community surveys. The first study to be reviewed is that of Saunders and Kershaw (1979) who introduced their study by acknowledging the growing amount of evidence which supports the existence of spontaneous remission from alcohol-related problems, and the difficulty that emerges when attempts are made to establish reliable spontaneous remission rates. Saunders and Kershaw are most interested in the social factors involved in the spontaneous remission process however: there 'appears to be a growing body of evidence which suggests that factors that exist within the social milieu of the alcoholic may be of more therapeutic importance than had previously been suspected' (1979: 253).

The evidence for the importance of social factors in the remission process to which they refer are studies by Bailey and Stewart (1966); Cahalan (1970); Knupfer (1972) and Edwards *et al.* (1977). The evidence provided by Bailey and Stewart (1966) was based on interviews with ninety-one respondents who had previously been identified as alcoholic in a household survey, and who were reinterviewed twice at two yearly intervals. At the first interview, thirteen respondents had modified their drinking patterns, but by the second interview, carried out four years after the initial contact, this number had fallen to six. Bailey and Stewart noted that none of the six had received psychiatric counselling, but attributed their improvement in drinking behaviour to the following factors: job change to less alcohol-related occupation (two men); improvement in marital relationship (two men); and serious physical illness (two men).

Cahalan's (1970) study of American problem drinkers discovered greater flexibility in drinking habits and the existence of different mechanisms in the process of spontaneous remission. Those problem drinkers who had previously increased their alcohol consumption attributed the rise in consumption to their increased ability to spend more money on alcohol, the influence of others, and having more time or opportunity to consume alcohol. In comparison to prior studies, relatively few problem drinkers attributed a rise in consumption to an attempt to use alcohol to reduce tension. The reasons cited by respondents who had decreased their alcohol consumption were also surprising when viewed from a disease model perspective. They included financial reasons, increased problems and responsibilities, having less need or desire to drink, becoming older or more mature, and health problems.

No mention was made in Cahalan's study of psychiatric treatment, AA or intensive psychotherapy as significant factors in bringing about remission from alcohol-related problems.

Knupfer's study (1972) was undertaken in San Francisco using data derived from two previous studies conducted in 1962 and 1964. Of the respondents who modified their drinking behaviours, less than 25 per cent had done so with the aid of treatment. Knupfer noted that significant life changes were more important than treatment, and marital and job changes were the most significant factors associated with spontaneous remission.

Saunders and Kershaw (1979) undertook a community survey to investigate the prevalence of alcohol-related problems on Clydeside. They identified 162 respondents who had alcohol-related problems in the past but were symptom free at the time of interview – out of a total sample of 3,600. Saunders and Kershaw hoped to discover the nature and duration of former problem drinking patterns and the major factors which the respondents believed had been most important in promoting their recovery. Of the original 162 respondents who were approached to be reinterviewed, 115 (71 per cent) complied, and their responses were analysed before being placed into one of the following four categories: questionnaire error (14 per cent); episodic over-consumers (32 per cent); problem drinkers (36 per cent); and definitely alcoholic (17 per cent). Two respondents were classed as still drinking problematically. The criteria used to define the category of problem drinker was to have had problems attributed to their alcohol consumption by either themselves or their family for a persistent period of not less than six months, and to have suffered problems in the areas of physical or psychological ill-health: 'and/or police, work and familial difficulties' (1979: 256).

The major criterion for the classification of a respondent as 'definitely alcoholic' was physical alcohol dependence, although other strict criteria also had to be met. The category of 'episodic over-consumers' contained respondents whom Saunders and Kershaw considered might be viewed as overly conscientious about their drinking, who had sustained only mild or no harm as a result of their drinking, which had usually been triggered by an extraordinary social occasion such as a wedding. This category was considered to consist of ordinary social drinkers, who were therefore used by Saunders and Kershaw as a control group.

The five most important causes of remission cited by the 'problem drinker' group were as follows: marriage (37 per cent); job change (32 per cent); physical illness (24 per cent); and family advice (12 per cent). The most important factors cited as reason for remission reported by the 'episodic over-consumers' ranked in declining order of importance were: job change; increased maturity; retirement; marriage and physical ill health. As Saunders and Kershaw observed, there is a marked similarity between the factors cited by both groups which primarily concern alterations in life circumstances.

It is significant that neither the 'problem drinkers' nor the 'episodic over-consumers' cited formal alcoholism treatment as the reason for their remission, although 7 per cent of 'problem drinkers' mentioned advice from a family doctor as a significant remission factor. The argument that 'problem drinking' is a problem for younger individuals, whereas 'alcoholism' (differentiated from the 'problem drinker' in terms of exhibiting greater severity of dependence) is a problem more associated with middle age, gains some support from this study. Saunders and Kershaw discovered that two-thirds of their problem drinking sample were aged under thirty at the time of their reported problem drinking, and the reasons for remission cited by those respondents over thirty and respondents below that age differed significantly (1979: 257).

Marriage was the most significant factor given for remission by those aged below thirty. At 30 years and above this factor was cited as important by only 7 per cent of the respondents, and although family influence was cited by an additional 14 per cent in this group it is clear that for older respondents ill health was the most important factor, being cited by 44 per cent of the sample. The only factor which appears to remain relatively stable in both age cohorts is a change in occupation to a job which is less alcohol-related.

Among the nineteen respondents classified as 'definitely alcoholic' only seven had received treatment, defined by Saunders and Kershaw as including visits to AA, Councils on Alcoholism and Alcohol Treatment Units, or receiving advice from any professional counselling service. The remaining twelve achieved remission without recourse to any treatment. However, when the mean duration of alcohol-related problems for those who received treatment was compared with those respondents who did not (19.7 years and 7.5 years respectively) the conclusion may be reached that spontaneous remission occurs most readily in less chronic cases (Saunders and Kershaw 1979: 259), indicating that formal treatment should perhaps be focused on individuals with a longer duration and greater severity of alcohol-related problems.

Marriage and job change scored equally as the factors which were most frequently advanced as being the cause of remission, indicating that even in the 'definitely alcoholic' category spontaneous remission factors are perhaps more important than treatment – a conclusion which directly contradicts the 'disease model' assumption that treatment is necessary if alcoholism is to be arrested.

Saunders and Kershaw also noted that even in those respondents who were defined as 'definitely alcoholic', eleven out of the twelve who received no treatment reported a return to regular drinking, although only one of the treated sample was classed as a regular drinker, the remaining six being abstinent. This difference between the treated and untreated 'definitely alcoholic' group could be attributed either to the exposure of the treated group to a treatment regime which demanded abstinence as a result of adherence to the disease model of alcoholism (see Heather and Robertson 1983: 76–7), or to an inability to continue drinking due to ill health. Saunders and Kershaw argue against an over simplistic reading of their results, as although the factors attributed to remission are reported individually, suggesting that marriage alone is the single most important factor, many respondents reported that their decision to marry overlapped with other events, such as the decision to leave an occupation which was alcohol-related or associated with heavy drinking. They argue that such a combination of factors was especially noticeable in younger problem drinkers and may lend support to Room's argument (1977) that problem drinking is culturally normal among young males, and should not therefore be considered deviant (Saunders and Kershaw 1979: 262).

In summary, Saunders and Kershaw make the following observations. First, spontaneous remission does occur in cases of alcohol dependence and major factors in the remission process are a new or improved marital relationship, which frequently coincides with leaving an occupation which offers access to alcohol or the opportunity to drink heavily. These factors taken together may be viewed as an increase in maturity. A process of 'maturing out' is therefore responsible for explaining remission from 'problem drinking' among primarily young men for whom such drinking may be culturally normal.

Second, treatment for alcohol-related problems may be most effective with older, long-standing cases of alcohol dependence, but even here successful treatment outcomes coincided with positive life changes which parallel those present in spontaneous remission. Those in treatment with the most severe cases of alcohol dependence were more likely to maintain abstinence as a long-term outcome, whereas less chronic cases were more likely to return to controlled drinking.

In 1981 Tuchfeld undertook a study of the factors involved in spontaneous remission as reported by thirty-five men and sixteen women living in the south-eastern states of America. Tuchfeld was satisfied that all fifty-one respondents had achieved remission from an alcohol-related problem without recourse to formal treatment – where formal treatment was defined as intervention by alcoholism treatment or rehabilitation centre, certain public or private psychiatric institutions, AA and similar voluntary organisations, certain psychological services, and persons trained in professional counselling or other therapeutic techniques.

All fifty-one respondents admitted to having social, physical or psychological problems related to alcohol use in the past. The prevalence of abstinence was much higher than in Saunders and Kershaw's study. Forty respondents were abstinent (78 per cent). One had returned to unguarded drinking, and ten to guarded or restrained drinking, where care was taken not to exceed a predetermined limit. Tuchfeld then analysed the data for factors which were associated with the decision to make an initial commitment to the resolution of drinking problems. The primary reasons for change and the number of respondents who reported them were as follows: personal illness or accident (seventeen); education in or educational material about alcoholism (six); religious conversion or experience (thirteen); direct intervention by immediate family (nine); direct intervention by friends (seven); financial problems created by drinking (eleven); alcohol-related death or illness of another person (seven); alcohol-related legal problems (four); extraordinary events including personal humiliation, exposure to negative role models, events during pregnancy, attempted suicide, and personal identity crises (fifteen).

Tuchfeld discovered an explicit rejection of the negative labels attached to the participants in formal drinking programmes. The label of 'alcoholism' or 'alcoholic' was found to be particularly stigmatising. Tuchfeld thought that the attitude of self-reliance exhibited by those who rejected formal treatment might coincide with a heightened receptivity to informal forms of social control, so that the help of friends and family would be acceptable as it could not be regarded as seeking formal treatment, which was categorically rejected by his sample of self-remitters. However, an initial commitment to changed drinking behaviour was not in itself sufficient to maintain change, unless this could be linked to what Tuchfeld referred to as 'maintenance factors'.

Maintenance factors involved a combination of social and psychological factors, none of which were sufficient on their own, but included 'social conditions – including the availability of non-alcohol-related leisure activities, reinforcement from family and friends, and the existence of relatively stable social and economic support systems' (Tuchfeld 1981: 636).

Lifestyle changes which incorporated participation in non alcohol-related activities seemed to be as important to the achievement of spontaneous remission, as did help from significant others. Tuchfeld also stressed the importance of objective social factors such as financial and employment stability. He presents a tentative model of the spontaneous remission process, which highlights the necessity of a combination of personal psychological factors such as a commitment to changing drinking behaviour, termed a 'moderator variable', which triggers a change in alcohol-related behaviour, which in turn is sustained by 'maintenance factors', such as support from significant others (informal social control) and 'objective social conditions' such as stability of employment.

Tuchfeld suggests that those who receive treatment follow the same form of remission pattern as those who do not, but the content of the process is different. Both groups undergo psychological changes in their attitude towards drinking, viewing it as less rewarding prior to altering their drinking behaviour. This change is then sustained by social controls. The person in treatment is assumed to accept and internalise as part of their self-concept the label of alcoholic, and is required to accept the institutionalised forces of social control. For the self-remitter, the stigmatising label of alcoholism is rejected and an individualised positive self image is constructed, which is supported by informal forms of social control such as employment status and familial support. Others who have studied the process of remission in relation to a number of addictive behaviours have also stressed the importance of making a firm commitment to change which must then be sustained by maintenance factors (Prochaska and DiClemente 1983; Klingemann 1991).

If many treatments are largely ineffective, or at least appear to be of unproven efficacy at the present time, this may reflect the failure of conventional alcoholism treatment to place sufficient emphasis on the importance of the positive and negative factors at work within the social milieu of their patients (Saunders and Allsop 1986). As Saunders and Allsop observed, this view is supported by the work of Moos and colleagues, who have undertaken a series of investigations into the post-treatment factors which were present or absent from the lives of 113 problem drinkers, followed up for two years after the end of their treatment (Billings and Moos 1983; Cronkite and Moos 1980; Moos *et al.* 1983). At the end of two years it was discovered that the number of former patients in remission equalled fifty-five, and that fifty-eight patients had relapsed.

Billings and Moos (1983) discovered three factors by which the two groups could be distinguished, apart from their drinking behaviour. First, patients who relapsed faced twice as many post-treatment negative life events as those in remission, but only half as many positive ones. Second, the preferred mode of coping utilised by the two groups differed: patients in remission tended to favour a cognitive behavioural approach to problem-solving, whereas the relapse group used problem avoidance, blamed others for problems, or relied on other drug use as coping strategies. Third, the availability and/or quality of available social resources differed significantly between the two groups, with the remission group enjoying greater family cohesion than the relapsers. As Saunders and Allsop point out, 'the characteristics associated with good outcome – such as familial cohesion, job satisfaction and the use of problem solving skills to counter adverse events, were not the consequence of abstinence but the facilitators of abstinence' (1986: 215).

Further evidence which supports the importance of social factors on treatment outcome can be found in the work of Azrin and colleagues (Hunt and Azrin 1973; Azrin 1976; Azrin *et al.* 1982). They restructured their clients' social environment by creating what they termed a Community Reinforcement Programme (CRA) (Hunt and Azrin 1973). The programme originally consisted of ensuring that their clients' social, marital and occupational functioning improved, but these improvements were contingent upon not drinking excessively. If extensive drinking occurred, the support of spouse, family and friends would be withdrawn in a predictable and consistent manner, only to be reinstated when drinking ceased, but without incurring recriminations for their previous drinking behaviour. To aid their clients' functioning, vocational training, assistance with job finding and even interviewing skills were provided. If the client was married and reconciliation with spouse and family were possible, intensive marital and family counselling were employed. If the client had no immediate family, a foster family consisting of more distant relatives or friends were requested to adopt the client, who would be encouraged to visit on a regular basis, but only on the understanding that if extensive drinking occurred then support would be withdrawn.

A 'social life' in the form of a self-financing group was established for the clients, to meet and share outings and other social pursuits: again attendance was only open to those who had not been drinking. The aim of using these instrumental learning techniques was to make the effects of drinking less desirable, and of non-drinking more desirable. The results of this experiment at the end of the first six months were that clients who received CRA spent only one sixth as much time drinking as the matched control group, who received alcohol education lectures and referral to AA, and the traditional hospital treatment.

Azrin (1976) reported the results of a second trial of the CRA versus a standard hospital programme, also working with alcohol dependent inpatients. The same counsellors were used to administer both programmes, but the most significant change to the CRA was the introduction of a disulfiram prescription and a disulfiram compliance programme. At the end of the six-month follow-up there was a remarkable difference between the two groups:

> the CRA clients showed fewer than 1 per cent drinking days per month, compared to 55 per cent in the control group; 20 per cent unemployment, compared to 56 per cent; and 7 per cent of days away from home, vs. 67 per cent in the traditional group.
>
> (Sisson and Azrin 1989: 253)

In 1982 Azrin et al. undertook an evaluation of the relative effectiveness of the different components of the CRA to assess the contribution made by the addition of disulfiram, by randomly assigning clients to one of three treatment groups. One group received traditional treatment, plus disulfiram which they were left to manage by themselves. The second group received traditional treatment, but in addition to disulfiram they also undertook the disulfiram compliance programme. The third treatment group received the complete spectrum of CRA components as outlined in Azrin (1976). The results of the full CRA programme were once again very impressive:

> At six month follow-up, the traditionally treated group reported over 50 per cent drinking days and about one third of their days unemployed and intoxicated. The Antabuse assurance procedures resulted in almost total sobriety for married or cohabiting clients, but had little effect for single people. The full CRA produced near total sobriety for all clients, married or single.
>
> (Sisson and Azrin 1989: 253)

Expenditure in terms of time, effort and resources are very high for this form of intervention, which make the adoption of such an approach on a large scale unlikely, while the choice of abstinence as the sole goal of treatment makes its use inappropriate for those seeking to control their drinking. However, as Miller and Hester noted, 'if one were to judge the effectiveness of alcoholism treatment methods based on the strength of scientific support available for them, the community reinforcement approach would surely be at the top of the list' (Miller and Hester 1986: 152).

It also clearly illustrates that the powerful forces inherent in the so-called 'spontaneous' remission process can be effectively utilised by the treatment professional, if in a more piecemeal manner.

PART TWO

The role of formal intervention in the remission process

In contrast to the scarcity of research literature which focuses specifically on the factors involved in the process of spontaneous remission from alcohol-related problems, the literature evaluating the effectiveness of different interventions is very extensive (Miller and Hester 1986). For this reason it has been necessary to restrict consideration to the five main reviews of the literature on treatment evaluation (Emrick 1975; Orford and Edwards 1977; Annis 1986; Miller and Hester 1986; Holder et al. 1991). These examine whether intensive treatments have demonstrated better treatment outcomes compared to interventions of brief duration, which can be utilised at lower cost.

In his review of treatment effectiveness, Emrick (1975) analysed 384 studies of psychologically oriented alcohol treatments in an attempt to answer two questions: first, whether a problem drinker's chances of improvement were enhanced by having one treatment rather than another; and, second, whether the improvement in drinking patterns was as strong or stronger with no formal treatment. Only those studies which had randomly assigned or adequately matched patient treatment groups were compared, in order to control for the influence of patient characteristics which might influence the treatment outcome. In addition, only those studies which reported a difference in outcome six months after the termination of treatment were compared, as Emrick claimed that differences in treatment outcome reported below that time interval were subject to high relapse rates, whereas by limiting analysis to 'differences found more than six months after treatment, conclusions could be based on stabilised data' (Emrick 1975: 90).

Emrick made a comparison of the effect of different treatment methods and reported the following conclusions. In thirty-one studies, no significant differences were reported in the effectiveness of the treatments compared. The remaining 353 reported significant differences between the various treatment groups. In all but five of these the differences could be attributed either to outcome evaluations based on observations made at a time interval of at most six months for at least one of the two groups being compared, or to one group remaining significantly longer in therapy than their comparison groups.

Emrick then compared the drinking outcome of untreated or minimally treated problem drinkers with more intensively treated problem drinkers in an attempt to discover if the duration of treatment had any bearing on abstinence or improvement outcomes. He noted that 13 per cent of the non-treated group were abstinent after at least six months and that 41 per cent had modified their drinking pattern – the results for the minimally treated group being 21 per cent abstinent and 43 per cent improved. Emrick was therefore able to suggest that '... many alcoholics can drink less or stop altogether with no or minimal treatment and (2) untreated alcoholics change as much as those receiving minimal treatment' (1975: 97).

The results of the comparison of untreated or minimally treated alcoholics with those receiving more intensive treatment showed no difference in abstinence rates between the three groups. Emrick summarises the results in the following manner:

> ... the findings suggest that alcoholics are, in a practical sense, as likely to stop drinking completely for six months or longer when they have no or minimal treatment as when they have more than the minimal treatment. On the other hand, treatment seems to increase an alcoholic's chances of at least reducing his drinking problems.
>
> (Emrick 1975: 97–8)

Emrick's optimistic view that treatment efforts have not been in vain has been criticised by Orford and Edwards (1977) and by Clare (1977). Orford and Edwards note that a clear conclusion on the relative effectiveness of treatment cannot be gained via a comparison between untreated or minimally treated alcoholics and those who receive more intensive treatment because this entails a comparison of individuals who have been refused treatment (or for whom treatment proved unsuitable), with patients who accepted treatment. Consequently, '... the bias induced by selective patient recruitment must vitiate Emrick's interpretation' (Orford and Edwards 1977: 19).

Orford and Edwards also argue that although Emrick was able to cite five suitably matched studies which may have suggested that one treatment regime resulted in achieving more improvement than those with which it was compared, the fact that thirty-one of the matched studies could find no such difference may have been the more significant result.

Further criticism concerned the methodology employed by three of the five studies in which Emrick claimed that one treatment was more effective. Detailed examination revealed problems over randomisation (Ends and Page 1957; Vogler *et al.* 1970) and attrition rates (Ends and Page 1957; Tomsovic and Edwards 1970; Vogler *et al.* 1970). Three of Emrick's five references to positive findings 'must therefore be seen as providing far from conclusive evidence' (Orford and Edwards 1977: 20).

Orford and Edwards undertook their own comparative study of the effectiveness of intensive treatment of alcohol dependence versus minimal intervention. One hundred couples where the male partner was diagnosed as alcohol dependent were carefully matched by intensive out-patient assessment of marital interaction and then randomly assigned either to an intensive treatment or to an advice-only group (N = 50 for each group). The advice-only group was given one counselling session and then left to work towards their stated drinking goals without further help, although they were free to seek additional treatment elsewhere. The intensive treatment group received 'a comprehensive programme of psychiatric and social work care' (Orford and Edwards 1977: xi).

The follow-up assessment consisted of an interview undertaken once every four weeks with wives only, and an intensive interview with both partners at the end of twelve months after the initial assessment. A further interview was undertaken at twenty-four months following treatment in an attempt to identify any evidence of controlled drinking. At the end of the first twelve months, complete data was available on forty-six out of the fifty advice-only group and forty-eight of the original fifty treatment group. A variety of treatment outcome measures were employed – including abstinence, consumption measures, the level of alcohol-related symptoms, hardship endured by wife, perceived improvement and employment stability. Using these criteria at the end of twelve months, Orford and Edwards concluded that there were no significant between-group differences.

As little compensatory treatment was sought by the advice-only group, the distinction between the group which received treatment and the group which did not remained fairly constant. There seemed to be no direct correlation in either group between the amount of treatment engaged in and the degree of improvement achieved, except that those members of the advice-only group who were more frequent attenders of AA meetings fared better than less frequent AA group attenders. A similar outcome was found in the treatment groups, where a better outcome was achieved by those who made more visits to their family doctor and to general hospitals than did less frequent attenders.

At the twelve month follow-up, Orford and Edwards asked their patients to identify the factors which seemed to have been the most important in aiding their improvement over the previous twelve months. Although formal treatment was accorded a place in the factors which positively affected outcome, it was ranked well below those factors which were deemed to be most important by both the intensive treatment and the advice-only groups. As Orford and Edwards note:

> in rank order, and for both groups, the four items given the highest ranking did not include in-patient care, out-patient care, AA, or other helping agency contact. Changes in external reality (especially occupation and housing), intrapsychic change, and change in the marital relationship were rated more highly.
>
> (1977: xii)

Orford and Edwards also noted that changes in external reality were likely to be valued more highly by the advice-only group than by the treatment group. This led them to conclude that although exposure to more intensive therapy failed to produce a more positive treatment outcome at twelve months, it succeeded in engaging patients in therapy and helped to modify their view of what had facilitated their improvement in drinking status. It is also significant that at the end of one year there was no significant correlation between the severity of alcohol-related symptoms endured by the patient and the differential effect of treatment or advice. It was not the 'more ill' patients (those with more 'symptoms' or 'troubles') who had done better with the treatment than advice (ibid.: xii).

This result would seem to contradict the view that treatment plays a necessary role in the remission of more severe cases of alcohol dependence, as even with these patients advice seems to have achieved a similar outcome to more intensive treatment. In a more recent study, Edwards and Taylor (1994) reanalysed the data from Orford and Edwards' original study to investigate whether more dependent patients achieve better treatment outcomes when exposed to more intensive treatment. The original findings were reconfirmed. They concluded: 'the robust finding appears to emerge that no three way interaction effect can be demonstrated between patient characteristics (including dependence), treatment intensity and outcome' (1994: 558).

In a review of the cost-effectiveness of inpatient treatment for alcohol dependence, Annis (1986) reported that on the basis of evidence from several randomised controlled trials (Willems *et al.*

1973; Page and Schaub 1979; Mosher *et al.* 1982), patients who received longer periods of hospitalisation failed to achieve more favourable treatment outcomes compared to patients hospitalised within the same institution for stays of brief duration. In addition, in two controlled studies (McLachlan and Stein 1982; Longabaugh et al. 1983), patients randomly assigned to receive hospital day care as opposed to inpatient treatment were found to achieve equal or better treatment outcomes.

Miller and Hester (1986) also reviewed the literature on the influence of setting and treatment intensity on treatment outcome. On the basis of twelve controlled studies they found no evidence to support the superiority of inpatient treatment over non-residential settings, and in five controlled studies which compared brief treatment with more intensive treatment they found less intensive methods provided better outcomes.

In an evaluation of the effects of treatment versus no treatment, it is perhaps unrealistic (as Orford and Edwards acknowledge) to attempt to study the effects of one treatment for longer than 12 months, since it becomes increasingly difficult to control for the effect of other help which may be sought as more time elapses. It is equally debatable whether we can gain more than a glimpse of the effectiveness of treatment in such a short time-scale, so perhaps it is only by studying the role of treatment via the greater time-scale afforded by longitudinal studies that the role which treatment plays in the remission process can be established. It is for this reason that we now turn in part three to the longitudinal evidence on the factors associated with remission from alcohol-related problems in both 'treated' and 'untreated' people with drinking problems.

PART THREE

Longitudinal studies of remission

The first attempt to study alcohol-related problems longitudinally was undertaken by Lemere (1953). Lemere sought information about the life course of 500 deceased alcoholics, as reported by their relatives who were Lemere's own psychiatric patients. While abstinence was achieved by 11 per cent of the sample by the time of death, mostly without recourse to formal treatment, and a further 3 per cent had returned to controlled drinking, the methodological adequacy of a study which relied completely on the memories of psychiatric patients could be called into question.

Kendell and Staton (1966) conducted a study into the outcome of fifty-seven alcoholics who rejected or were refused treatment by the Maudsley Hospital in London between May 1950 and June 1961. This sample was followed up for between two and thirteen years, and their outcomes compared with a similar study of treated alcoholics (Wing 1956). At the final follow-up, 18 per cent had died, 8 per cent as a result of suicide. Of the remainder, 11 per cent returned to controlled drinking, and a further 20 per cent achieved stable abstinence (Kendell and Staton 1966).

In 1968 Drew published an important paper which suggested the possibility of alcoholism as a self-limiting disease. This conception of alcoholism was based on a study of demographic data for the Australian state of Victoria, in which a direct comparison was made between the incidence and prevalence of alcohol-related problems for the year 1963. Drew discovered that instead of the predictive prevalence being equal to the accumulated incidence of alcohol dependence – which should have been the case for an irreversible condition with low mortality rates – the actual rate of prevalence for alcohol dependence began to steadily decline after the age of 40. Drew noted that all but two of the studies published world-wide, confirmed that after a peak age of between 40 and 50 years, the prevalence of alcoholism in older age cohorts declined.

Drew offered three possible hypotheses for the declining prevalence of alcoholism after the age of 50. The first hypothesis, which he partially accepted, was that many alcoholics aged 50 or above had died or become institutionalised as a result of acute alcoholic psychosis, suicidal gestures, or fatal road accidents. The second hypothesis, that treatment was responsible for the decline in the prevalence of alcoholism, he rejected on the basis of studies which questioned the effectiveness of treatment (Gerard *et al.* 1966; Rossi *et al.* 1963; Kendall and Staton 1966). The third hypothesis, that the prevalence of alcoholism declines with age, received the greatest support, and he observed that the chances of achieving remission from alcoholism increased for individuals aged over 40. Drew commented:

increasing maturity and responsibility, decreasing drive, increasing social withdrawal, changing social pressures, reduced financial resources, and onset of psychiatric disturbance, are factors which often accompany ageing and which may contribute to this reduction of alcohol problems with increasing age.

(Drew 1968: 964–5)

On the basis of this study, Drew concluded that 'alcoholism tends to disappear with increasing age. Although morbidity and mortality may account for a large part, a significant proportion of this disappearance is probably due to spontaneous recovery' (Drew 1968: 965).

Vaillant (1983) argues that in coming to this conclusion, Drew had given insufficient consideration to the alternative explanation that a high mortality rate, rather than spontaneous remission, was responsible for the declining prevalence of alcoholism in older age cohorts. High mortality as an explanation is supported by Lemere (1953), and is consistent with the view of alcoholism held by Jellinek (1952). To investigate the strength of this alternative hypothesis, Vaillant undertook his own review of ten longitudinal studies of the natural history of alcohol-related problems.

Each study Vaillant reviewed lasted a minimum of seven years. Because of the time-scale, those who were initially untreated may have been exposed to a variety of treatments over time, making it futile to attempt to maintain a distinction between treated and untreated groups. Vaillant noted, however, that a positive relationship existed between the length of follow-up and a high remission rate. A longer follow-up period seemed to be a more reliable predictor of a high remission rate than was exposure to treatment: 'the implication is that alcoholics recover not because we treat them, but because they heal themselves' (1983: 126).

Of the ten studies reviewed by Vaillant, that by Goodwin *et al.* (1971) contained the youngest sample, with an average age of 27 years. This study also reported the highest rate of return to asymptomatic drinking amongst a non-treatment seeking population. The reasons for remission which were most commonly reported by Goodwin's respondents were marriage and increased family responsibilities. Vaillant had a similar finding for his core city sample, who were aged between 20 and 30 years.

Further confirmation came from Ojesjo's study (1981), in which 32 per cent of the sample had achieved abstinence or remission at the end of a 15-year follow-up period. The factors which were identified as being predictive of a poor prognosis were, in rank order: severity of alcohol involvement; age; work; poor interpersonal relations. The predictors of a good prognosis were: 'the ability to abstain from alcohol, emotional and social stability, and particularly a satisfactory combination of work and interpersonal adaptation' (1981: 398).

In concluding his analysis of these ten longitudinal studies, Vaillant observed that the two studies which reported the highest remission rates (his own core city sample and that of Sundby 1967) incorporated a time interval for follow-up which was double that of the other longitudinal studies. He summarised: 'Drew's hypothesis that eventually alcoholics recover appears at least partly vindicated, and the natural rate of stable remission from alcoholism is perhaps 2 to 3 per cent a year' (Vaillant 1983: 128).

Fillmore (1987a) conducted an analysis of two North American longitudinal general population samples in order to demonstrate that changes in the incidence, chronicity and remission patterns of heavy drinking and alcohol-related problems are age-related for American men. She concluded that the 'incidence of heavy drinking and alcohol problems decreases with age and that the chronicity of alcohol problems is highest in the middle years of life' (1987a: 81).

In a further study, Fillmore analysed data from a longitudinal general population sample to describe patterns of drinking at each decade across the adult life-course for women. These patterns were then compared with those of men in the sample. For most decades, the incidence of men drinking at a level which could place them at risk of health or social problems exceeded that of women, although the sex ratio for drinking problems nearly converges in the thirties. The convergence was short lived, and in their 40s, men exceed women in all drinking incidence measures, suggesting that women's alcohol disorders have a shorter duration than those of men (Fillmore 1987b).

Self reported and contingent factors associated with remission

In *The Natural History of Alcoholism* Vaillant (1983) addressed the question of which self-reported and contingent factors were most important in helping alcoholics attain abstinence or a return to asymptomatic drinking. His findings were based on information obtained from his own longitudinal analysis of 456 under-privileged Boston men followed up for approximately 40 years (the core city sample). Vaillant observed no difference in the frequency of treatment visits or in the severity of alcohol-related problems between those who were currently abstinent and those who continued drinking. Respondents were asked what had been important to achieving abstinence, and what had been tried but failed. Among those who had been abstinent for at least one year, only 30 per cent cited treatment as being a significant factor.

Psychotherapy was found to be ineffective for all the core city problem drinkers who received it, and although a greater percentage of the upper-middle class sample received psychotherapy than did the core city sample (62 per cent as opposed to 8 per cent), only two individuals reported that psychotherapy had aided remission.

The evidence from longitudinal surveys lends powerful support to the conclusions drawn from studies of treatment effectiveness reviewed in part two of this chapter. Thus Bailey and Stewart (1966), Knupfer (1972) and Saunders and Kershaw (1979) all found ill-health, job change and improvement in marital relationships to be important, while respondents in Orford and Edwards' (1977) study cited changes in external circumstances – especially housing and job change – intrapsychic changes and improved marital relationships, as being more important than formal treatment. Tuchfeld (1981) and Moos *et al.* (1983) also emphasised the significance of social support. It is safe to conclude that changes in the social and physical environment have been shown to be at least as important in securing the attainment of long-term remission from alcohol-related problems as access or exposure to treatment:

> the most important single prognostic variable associated with remission among alcoholics who attend alcohol clinics is having something to lose if they continue to abuse alcohol. Not only do alcoholics with stable jobs and stable marriages have the

most to lose; they also enjoy the best social supports, and thus are more closely supervised.

(Vaillant 1983: 191)

Improvements in the social milieu of the client appear to be extremely important in securing remission from alcohol-related problems. Social workers already possess many of the skills which are necessary to deliver an effective service to problem drinking clients (Leckie 1990). If helping clients who have problems with drug and alcohol use is to be accorded a higher priority as part of the movement towards providing care in the community, with further training social workers should be able to make a valuable contribution towards meeting this objective.

REFERENCES

Abel, P. (1983) *Alcohol-Related Problems in Social Work Caseloads*, Bristol: Social Services Department, Avon County Council.

Annis, H. M. (1986) 'Is inpatient rehabilitation of the alcoholic cost effective? Con Position', in B. Stimmel (ed.) *Controversies in Alcoholism and Substance Abuse*, New York: Haworth Press.

Azrin, N. (1976) 'Improvements in the community-reinforcement approach to alcoholism', *Behaviour Research and Therapy*, 14: 339–48.

Azrin, N., Sisson, R., Meyers, R. and Godley, M. (1982) 'Alcoholism treatment by disulfiram and community-reinforcement therapy', *Journal of Behavioural Therapy and Experimental Psychiatry*, 13: 105–12.

Bailey, M. and Stewart, J. (1966) 'Normal drinking by persons reporting previous problem drinking', *Quarterly Journal of Studies on Alcohol*, 28: 305–15.

Billings, A. and Moos, R. (1983) 'Psychosocial processes of recovery among alcoholics and their families: implications for clinicians and programme evaluators', *Addictive Behaviours*, 8: 205–18.

Bratfos, O. (1974) *The Course of Alcoholism: Drinking, Social Adjustment and Health*, Oslo: Universitet Forlaget.

Cahalan, D. (1970) *Problem Drinkers*, San Francisco: Jossey Bass.

Clancy, J. (1961) 'Outpatient treatment of the alcoholic', *Journal of the Iowa State Medical Society*, 29: 956–67.

Clancy, J., Vornbrock., R. and Vanderhoof, E. (1965) 'Treatment of alcoholics: a follow-up study', *Diseases of the Nervous System*, 26: 555–61.

Clare, A. W. (1977) 'How good is treatment?' in G. Edwards and M. Grant (eds) *Alcoholism: New Knowledge and New Responses*, London: Croom Helm.

Costello, R. M. (1975) 'Alcoholism treatment and evaluation, II: collation of two year follow-up studies', *International Journal of Addiction*, 10: 857–67.

Cronkite, R. and Moos, R. (1980) 'The determinants of post-treatment functioning of alcoholic patients: a conceptual framework', *Journal of Consulting and Clinical Psychology*, 48: 305–16.

Davies, I. and Raistrick, D. (1981) *Dealing with Drink: Helping Problem Drinkers, a Handbook*, London: British Broadcasting Corporation.

Drew, L. R. H. (1968) 'Alcoholism as a self-limiting disease', *Quarterly Journal of Studies on Alcohol*, 29: 956–67.

Edwards, G., Orford, J., Egert, S., Hawker, A., Kensman, C., Mitcheson, M., Oppenheimer, E. and Taylor, C. (1977) 'Alcoholism: a controlled trial of "treatment" and "advice"', *Journal of Studies on Alcohol*, 38(5): 1004.

Edwards, G. and Taylor, C., (1994) 'A test of the matching hypothesis: alcohol dependence, intensity of treatment and 12 month outcome', *Addiction*, 89 (5): 553–61.

Emrick, C. D. (1975) 'A review of psychologically oriented treatment of alcoholism: II the relative effectiveness of different treatment approaches and the effectiveness of treatment versus no treatment', *Journal of Studies on Alcohol*, 36: 88–108.

Ends, E. J. and Page, C. W. (1957) 'A study of three types of group psychotherapy with hospitalised male inebriates', *Quarterly Journal of Studies on Alcohol*, 18: 263–77.

Eysenck, H. and Beech, R. (1971) 'Counter conditioning and related methods', in A. Bergin and S. Garfield (eds) *Handbook of Psychotherapy and Behaviour Change: An Empirical Analysis*, New York: Wiley.

Fillmore, K. M. (1987a) 'Prevalence, incidence and chronicity of drinking patterns and problems among men as a factor of age: a longitudinal and cohort analysis', *British Journal of Addiction*, 82(1): 77–83.

Fillmore, K. M. (1987b) 'Women's drinking across the adult life course as compared to men's', *British Journal of Addiction*, 82(7): 801–11.

Gerard, D. L., Saenger, G. and Wile, R. (1966) 'The abstinent alcoholic', *Archives of General Psychiatry*, 6: 83–95.

Glaser, F. B. and Ogbourne, A. C. (1982) 'Does A.A. really work?' *British Journal of Addiction*, 77: 123–30.

Goodwin, D. W., Crane, J. B. and Guze, S. B. (1971) 'Felons who drink: an 8-year follow-up', *Quarterly Journal of Studies on Alcohol*, 32: 136–47.

Heather, N. and Robertson, I. (1983) *Controlled Drinking*, London: Methuen.

Heather, N. and Robertson, I. (1985) *Problem Drinking: The New Approach*, London: Penguin.

Hebblethwaite, D. (1979) 'Alcohol problems, social work's response and responsibility', *Social Work Today*, 10 (31): 8–11.

Holder, H., Longabaugh, R., Miller, W. R. and Rubonis, A. V. (1991) 'The cost effectiveness of treatment for alcoholism: a first approximation', *Journal of Studies on Alcohol*, 52 (6): 517–40.

Hunt, G. and Azrin, N. (1973) 'A community-reinforcement approach to alcoholism', *Behaviour Research and Therapy*, 14: 339–48.

Isaacs, J. and Moon, G. (1985) *Alcohol Problems: The Social Work*

Response, SSRIU Report 13, Social Services Research and Intelligence Unit: Hampshire Social Services Department.

Jellinek, E. M. (1952) 'Phases of alcohol addiction', *Quarterly Journal of Studies on Alcohol*, 13: 673–84.

Jellinek, E. M. (1960) *The Disease Concept of Alcoholism*, New Haven: Hillhouse Press.

Jessor, R. (1985) 'Adolescent problem drinking: psychosocial aspects and developmental outcome', in L. Towle (ed.) *Proceedings from NIAAA – WHO Collaborating Center Designation Meeting and Alcohol Research Seminar*, Washington DC.

Kendell, R. E. and Staton, M. C. (1966) 'The fate of untreated alcoholics', *Quarterly Journal of Studies on Alcohol*, 27: 30–41.

Kissin, B., Rosenblatt, S. M. and Machover, S. (1968) 'Prognostic factors in alcoholism', *Psychiatric Research Report*, 24: 22–43.

Klingemann, H. K. (1991) 'The motivation for change from problem alcohol and heroin use', *British Journal of Addiction*, 86 (6): 727–44.

Knupfer, G. C. (1972) 'Ex-problem drinkers', in M. Roff, L. Robins and H. Pollack (eds) *Life History Research in Psychopathology*, vol. 2, Minneapolis: University of Minnesota Press.

Kreitman, N. (1977) 'Three themes in the epidemiology of alcoholism', in G. Edwards and M. Grant (eds) *Alcoholism: New Knowledge and New Responses*, London: Croom Helm.

Leckie, T. (1990) 'Social work and alcohol', in S. Collins (ed.) *Alcohol, Social Work and Helping*, London: Routledge.

Leckie, T., Osborn, A. and Grimes, A. (1984) 'Alcoholics: too anonymous?' *Social Work Today*, 16(4): 16–17.

Lemere, F. (1953) 'What happens to alcoholics?' *American Journal of Psychiatry*, 109: 674–76.

Longabaugh, R., McCrady, B., Fink, E., Stout, R., McAuley, T., Doyle, C. and McNeill, D. (1983) 'Cost effectiveness of alcoholism treatment in partial versus inpatient settings: six month outcomes', *Journal of Studies on Alcohol*, 44: 1049–71.

McCrady, B. S. (1991) 'Promising but under-utilized treatment approaches', *Alcohol Health and Research World*, 15 (3): 215–18.

McLachlan, J. F. C. and Stein, R. L. (1982) 'Evaluation of a day clinic for alcoholics', *Journal of Studies on Alcohol*, 42: 261–72.

Miller, W. R. (ed.) (1980) *The Addictive Behaviours: Treatment of Alcoholism, Drug Abuse, Smoking and Obesity*, Oxford: Pergamon Press.

Miller, W. R. and Hester, R. K. (1980) 'Treating the problem drinker: modern approaches', in W. R. Miller (ed.) *The Addictive Behaviours: Treatment of Alcoholism, Drug Abuse, Smoking and Obesity*, Oxford: Pergamon Press.

Miller, W. R. and Hester, R. K. (1986) 'The effectiveness of alcoholism treatment: what research reveals', in W. R. Miller and N. Heather (eds) *Treating Addictive Behaviours: Processes of Change*, London: Plenum Press.

Moos, R., Cronkite, R. and Finney, J. (1983) 'A conceptual framework for alcoholism treatment evaluation', in E. M. Pattison and E.

Kaufman (eds) *Encyclopaedic Handbook of Alcoholism*, New York: Gardiner Press.

Mosher, V., Davies, J., Mulligan, D. and Iber, F. L. (1982) 'Comparison in outcome in a nine day and a thirty day alcoholism treatment program', *Journal of Studies on Alcohol*, 43: 261–72.

Mulford, H. (1978) *Accelerating the natural alcoholic recovery process.* Paper presented at the 32nd International Conference on Alcohol and Drug Abuse, Warsaw: Poland.

Myerson, D. J. and Mayer, J. (1966) 'Origins, treatment and destiny of Skid Row alcoholic men', *New England Journal of Medicine*, 275: 419–24.

Ojesjo, L. (1981) 'Long-term outcome in alcohol abuse and alcoholism among males in the Lundy general population, Sweden', *British Journal of Addiction*, 76 (4): 391–400.

Orford, J. (1985) *Excessive Appetites: A Psychological View of Addictions*, Chichester: Wiley.

Orford, J. and Edwards, G. (1977) *Alcoholism*, Maudsley Monograph No. 26, Oxford: Oxford University Press.

Page, R. D. and Shaub, L. B. (1979) 'Efficacy of a three- versus a five-week alcohol treatment program', *International Journal of the Addictions*, 14: 697–714.

Pittman, D. J. and Tate, R. C. (1972) 'A comparison of two treatment programs for alcoholics', *International Journal of Social Psychiatry*, 18: 183–93.

Prochaska, J. and DiClemente, C. (1983) 'Stages and processes of self-change in smoking', *Journal of Consulting and Clinical Psychology*, 51: 390–95.

Raistrick, D. and Davidson, R. (1985) *Alcoholism and Drug Addiction*, London: Churchill Livingstone.

Robson, R. A. H., Paulus, I. and Clarke, G. G. (1965) 'An evaluation of the effect of a clinical treatment program on the rehabilitation of alcoholic patients', *Quarterly Journal of Studies on Alcohol*, 26: 264–78.

Roizen, R., Cahalan, D. and Shanks, P. (1978) 'Spontaneous remission among untreated problem drinkers', in D. B. Kandel (ed.) *Longitudinal Research on Drug Use: Empirical Findings and Methodological Issues*, Washington: Hemisphere Publishing Corporation.

Room, R. (1977) 'Measurement and distribution of drinking patterns and problems in general populations', in G. Edwards, M. Gross, M. Keller, R. Moser and R. Room (eds) *Alcohol Related Disabilities*, Geneva: World Health Organisation.

Rossi, J. J., Stach, A. and Bradley, N. J. (1963) 'Effects of treatment of male alcoholics in a mental hospital; a follow-up study', *Quarterly Journal of Studies on Alcohol*, 13: 673–84.

Royal College of Psychiatrists (1979) *Alcohol and Alcoholism: The Report of a Special Committee of The Royal College of Psychiatrists*, London: Tavistock.

Saunders, W. and Allsop, S. (1986) 'Giving up addictions', in F. Watts (ed.) *New Developments in Clinical Psychology*, Chichester: Wiley.

Saunders, W. and Kershaw, P. (1979) 'Spontaneous remission from alcoholism – a community study', *British Journal of Addiction*, 74: 251–65.
Shaw, S., Cartwright, A., Spratley, T. and Harwin, J. (1978) *Responding
to Drink Problems*, London: Croom Helm.
Sisson, W. R. and Azrin, N. H. (1989) 'The community reinforcement
approach', in R. K. Hester and W. R. Miller (eds) *Handbook of
Alcoholism Treatment Approaches*, Oxford: Pergamon Press.
Sobell, M. B. and Sobell, L. C. (1973) 'Alcoholics treated by individu-
alised behaviour therapy: one-year treatment outcome', *Behaviour,
Research and Therapy*, 11: 599–618.
Sundby, P. (1967) *Alcoholism and Mortality*, Oslo: Universitet Forlaget.
Tomsovic, M. and Edwards, R. V. (1970) 'Lysergide treatment of schiz-
ophrenic and non-schizophrenic alcoholics: a controlled evaluation',
Quarterly Journal of Studies on Alcohol, 31: 932–49.
Tuchfeld, B. S. (1981) 'Spontaneous remission in alcoholics: empirical
observation and theoretical implications', *Journal of Studies on
Alcohol*, 42 (7): 626–41.
Vaillant, G. E. (1983) *The Natural History of Alcoholism*, London:
Harvard University Press.
Voetglin, W. L. and Broz, A. (1949) 'The conditioned reflex treatment
of chronic alcoholism, X: an analysis of 3,125 admissions over a period
of ten and a half years', *Annals of Internal Medicine*, 30: 580–97.
Vogler, R. E., Lunde, S. E., Johnson, G. R. and Martin, P. L. (1970)
'Electrical aversion conditioning with chronic alcoholics', *Journal of
Consulting Clinical Psychology*, 34: 302–7.
Willems, P. J. A., Letemendia, F. J. J. and Arroyave, F. (1973) 'A two year
follow-up study comparing short and long stay inpatient treatments
of alcoholics', *British Journal of Psychiatry*, 122: 637–48.
Wing, J. K. (1956) 'A four year follow-up of 50 alcohol addicts after treat-
ment in hospital'. Unpublished PhD thesis, London University.
Yates, F. E. and Norris, H. (1981) 'The use made of treatment: an alter-
native approach to the evaluation of alcoholism services', *New
Directions in the Study of Alcohol*, 31: 932–49.

Chapter 7

Gender divisions and drinking problems

Jan Waterson

INTRODUCTION

Women's drinking is paradoxical. Women of all ages drink less than men and consequently experience fewer alcohol related problems (Plant 1990; Goddard 1991; OPCS 1992; WHO 1992; McDonald 1994). It is very difficult to gain an accurate estimate of the extent of women's alcohol-related problems. Although we have some figures (albeit now dated) for numbers in Alcohol Treatment Units, where the ratio of female to male patients declined from 1:3 in 1968 to 1:2 by 1980 (Beory and Merry 1986), these figures are likely to be the tip of the iceberg. For as Thom describes in Chapter 8, women face formidable barriers to treatment. Furthermore, these treatment figures do not take into account women receiving help from other specialist counselling agencies, social services or other parts of the health service, including GPs. Indeed, it is now established that a sizable proportion of patients who are treated by a wide range of medical specialities, in particular emergency services and orthopaedics, are likely to have alcohol problems (Cherpital 1994).

In terms of other possible indicators of alcohol-related problems, women are only responsible for 5 per cent of all drinking and driving offences, but between 1975 and 1989 the number of offences committed by females per 100,000 drivers increased by 65 per cent – at a time when the proportion of male offences was decreasing. Similarly rates for liver cirrhosis have been increasing amongst women. Significantly, women are only responsible for 7 per cent of all drunkenness offences, but those that are heavy drinkers are more likely to be victims of violence, abuse and crime (Fillmore 1985a).

The reliability of national data on drinking patterns is questionable. Even amongst those people that surveys do reach it is known that heavier drinkers tend to underestimate their consumption. Nevertheless interesting trends emerge.

Recent national data show that rates of drinkers as compared with non-drinkers are converging between the sexes (Goddard 1991). The 1990 GHS indicates that women are twice as likely as men to be non-drinkers (12 per cent to 6 per cent) and are much less likely to drink above sensible levels (11 per cent to 28 per cent) (OPCS 1992). The current sensible drinking level advocated for women is less than fourteen units per week. Consumption in excess of this is deemed to be potentially harmful. Women drinking 35 units or more a week are very likely to suffer liver damage and other physical problems (Royal College of General Practitioners 1986). For men the sensible limit is 21 units per week.

Amongst women heavier drinking is associated with socioeconomic status. In 1990, 14 per cent of professional women were drinking more than the sensible limits, whereas only 6 per cent of the women in the unskilled manual group were drinking at these levels (OPCS 1992).

As common sense might suggest, heavy drinking is more common amongst younger women (under 25 years) compared with older women (over 65) (17 per cent to 5 per cent). Young women who are separated, divorced or widowed seem to be a particularly vulnerable group. One-quarter are drinking above sensible limits, and an increasing and worrying number of them are consuming dangerous levels of thirty-six or more units a week. In general, single women are more likely than married women to drink more than fourteen units a week (14 per cent to 11 per cent). Estimates suggest that lesbian women are particularly at risk of alcohol problems. Amongst married women (aged 25 to 44) those with dependent children drank less than those without children (10 per cent to 33 per cent).

Average consumption among women is increasing, and heavy drinking (more than 14 units per week) is slowly but steadily rising (OPCS 1992). Although they are more susceptible to physical damage than men (Department of Health and Royal College of General Practitioners 1992), women who have drinking problems have, in general, not been catered for adequately by helping agencies (DAWN 1988; Waterson and Ettorre 1989; Coupe 1992; DAWN 1994).

One indicator of the health of any research field might be a measure of the volume of publications emanating from that particular speciality. Whilst in no way suggesting that volume is necessarily linked to quality, it remains an indicator of interest and typicality. Until 1980 little was written on the general topic of women and alcohol from either a medical, epidemiological or social perspective. Between 1929 and 1970 only twenty-eight English language papers were written (see Lisansky 1957). In 1972 Lindbeck was able to write: 'the woman alcoholic has been a step-child in the field of research. References to her problem are abundant, but concentrated focus on her is comparatively rare' (1972: 567).

Since then interest has grown, starting in the US and later developing in the UK. Several major literature reviews were produced in the 1980s (e.g. Kalant 1980; Shaw 1980) and interest is now well established (Bailey 1990; Plant 1990; Department of Health and Royal College of General Practitioners 1992; WHO 1992; Ettorre 1992).

In much of the literature, female drinking has, until recently, been stigmatised and viewed as essentially unfeminine (Ettorre 1992). Such a perspective, which views women's drinking as due to individual irresponsibility and ignorance (reinforced should they be pregnant), is not new. Reports highlighting the dangers of drinking during pregnancy have frequently cited historical sources to support their case. In fact, far from presenting the historical pedigree of their arguments such quotations simply serve to illustrate that double standards for women as compared to men have a long history. Indeed, concern about female problem drinking has tended to be heightened at times of rapid change in women's roles: at the turn of the century and in the 1970s. Given that such changes threatened established gender relations it is no accident that existing research has concentrated on potential damage to the foetus rather than any impact on women themselves, and that faulty sex-role performance is so frequently referred to in the literature on women's drinking that it has almost become a governing image. The next section of this chapter briefly traces the development of this image.

A critique of these perspectives follows, and an alternative view which stresses the importance of gender and socioeconomic position is given. This is based on empirical data, drawn from an interview study of sixty female alcohol users who did not have identified problems, and who had recently become mothers for the first time (Waterson 1992). The data will be used to demonstrate that conventional interpretations not only ignore the 'gendering' of alcohol as a social problem, but also discount the vital importance of social advantage or disadvantage in both structuring the opportunities to drink and in creating stresses which might encourage drinking.

DOUBLE STANDARDS AND THE NEED TO CONTROL FEMALE DRINKING

Much of the discourse about female drinking has implied a double standard. Drinking has traditionally been viewed as a legitimate male pursuit, inappropriate for females. A useful aside may be given here. Berridge and Edwards (1981) note that concern about opiate use first centred around middle-class female use for enjoyment. This at the very least suggests that social concern about the use of some potentially addictive substances increases when they are used for female pleasure. Certainly in the ancient world alcohol was regarded as a female aphrodisiac – and Biblical and Classical references probably refer to a male attempt to control female behaviour (Abel 1984). The Romans at one time and the Jews in the post-Biblical era forbade women to drink alcohol at all.

Such double standards have been amplified by the notion that as drinking is inappropriate for females, those that persist in drinking heavily for whatever reason must in some way be intrinsically flawed as females (Blume 1991). Historical examples graphically illustrate this contrast. William Hogarth's print 'Gin Lane' of 1751 depicts many of the evils attributable to female gin drinking: early death, drunkenness, and child neglect. This is in direct contrast to another of his engravings 'Beer Street', which illustrates the health and well-being of male drinking. In the late nineteenth century Darwinian ideas of heredity and the development of statistical science encouraged studies correlating the birth of imbeciles with parental drinking. A prison physician surveyed the 600 offspring of 120 alcoholic women in a Liverpool prison in 1899 and wrote:

> We are familiar with the fact that the chronic alcoholism of one or both parents appears as the first moment in the degenerative career of a whole family. . . . In suppressing the female

drunkard the community not only eliminates an element always individually useless and constantly liable to become individually noxious, it also prevents the procreation of children under the conditions most apt to render them subsequently, if they survive, a burden or a danger to society.

(Sullivan 1899: 499)

Despite his apparent concern with the reproductive capacity of both parents, it is noteworthy that he makes a point of singling out the female drunkard for considerable censure.

Public interest in drinking has always centred around control, but it does seem that at times of economic or social crisis a particular ideology of the feminine role becomes part of the repertoire of that public control. Certainly scare tactics, such as suggestions that their reproductive organs would wither and perish, were used against the suffragettes, and more recently juvenile delinquency and mental breakdown have been blamed on the supposed decline of motherhood – without adequate empirical justification (Ferrence 1980).

There have been two distinct periods of heightened interest in women's drinking – the turn of this century and the 1970s and early 1980s. Both were times of major social and political change, including changes in women's roles with respect to the State, the labour market and the domestic realm (McDowall 1989). The first was marked by the struggle for emancipation and the second by the 1960s women's movement (Rowbotham 1990). At both times public anxiety about the potential decline of motherhood spilled over into other areas including women's drinking.

Although there is long-standing evidence of the existence of double standards, until the late nineteenth century public interest had largely centred on male drinking, which was seen as potentially detrimental to industrial productivity and the family. Indeed, early suffrage movements allied with the Temperance campaign! However, towards the end of the last century there was a discernible shift of concern to the importance of the mother as the core of the family system, safeguarding the well-being of husband and children alike and preserving the moral order of the family (Lewis 1986, 1991). In this way the double standard became part of an ideology. Despite contemporary socialist emphasis on chronic drinking as a reaction to intolerable conditions and poverty, in the public consciousness, heavy female drinking was linked with poor childbearing capacities and prostitution. This concern was not confined to Britain. During the 1890s there was even talk of compulsory sterilisation of inebriate women in Imperial Germany, though this was never implemented (Vogt 1984). In an age amply endowed with moralistic fervour it was natural that the sins of the parents, especially mothers, could only too easily be seen to be bestowed upon the children.

In addition, a new awareness of the long-established custom of working-class females drinking in pubs was emerging and being documented. The 1899 Royal Commission on Licensing Laws had drawn attention to the plight of the children of drunken parents. In 1900 Rowntree and Sherwall, prominent social reformers, suggested that female alcoholism had doubled in the previous twenty years in a pamphlet entitled 'The Temperance Problem and Social Reform' (see Gutzke 1984). In the ensuing debates, widespread fears about a rising tide of female insobriety were provoked. At the same time the experience of the Boer War had exposed the poor health of many of the recruits to armed forces. Serious concern about these revelations, and anxiety about high infant mortality rates against the background of a declining birth rate provided a fertile seed-bed for a focus on this apparent problem of female drinking. Public concern became focused on how to improve the physical well-being of the population (Lewis 1980).

At the time alcoholism was viewed as a degenerative condition – consequently maternal alcoholism came to be viewed as a major obstacle to improving the nation's health. A well-orchestrated campaign against female drinking was carried out between 1899 and 1907 (Gutzke 1984). In 1903 the first articles appeared linking maternal alcoholism with weakness in the offspring and hence in the whole population – threatening the nation and eventually the empire. Such concern can be interpreted as an attempt to control the apparent threat of women's widening roles and demand for the franchise, to the symbolic bulwarks of the nation, the family, marriage and property rights. After all, the symbol of respectability in Edwardian England was that a man should be able to 'keep' his wife (Lewis 1986, 1991). That female drinking was seen as a symbolic threat and a stigmatised activity was clearly shown by the higher percentage of female as compared with male drunkards who were incarcerated in inebriate reformatories in the early part of the century (Hunt 1988). Further evidence comes from this short extract from *Life and Labour of the People of London*, written in 1902 by Charles Booth.

> The increase in drinking is to be laid mainly to the account of the female sex. This latter phase seems to be one of the unexpected results of the emancipation of woman. On the one hand she has become more independent of man, industrially and financially, and on the other more of a comrade than before, and in neither capacity does she feel any shame at entering a public house. ... All around London are growing up suburbs of such houses whose occupants have just enough to live on comfortably. Women are left at home, small ailments, the immediate stimulus of drink, that is how it begins.
>
> (Booth 1902: 59)

The earlier, late nineteenth century image of uncontrollable, rebellious, urban working-class female drinking is here extended into a new concept of the suburban woman lacking in male supervision.

In an effort to control female drinking, the 1908 Children's Act excluded children under fourteen years of age from public houses for the first time. Gutzke has interpreted this legislation as follows:

> It can be seen as part of the Edwardian response to disturbing social changes, reflecting upper and middle-class fears not only of an alien and threatening working-class culture, but of women's changing role in society. Apprehensions over female inebriety derived partially from an inability to accept women's greater freedom outside the home – a motive detected by historians who have explored the alleged incompetence of working wives. Legislators, doctors and social investigators were often concerned not so much that diminished restraint in entering pubs would lead to correspondingly greater drunkenness as that women's higher status was a threat to the family, evident in declining birth rates, marriage property rights and suffrage demands.
>
> (Gutzke 1984: 80)

Moving to the second identified period of interest, between 1970 and 1986 over 3,000 papers on the effects of alcohol on pregnancy were added to the world literature, far surpassing in quantity all other work on women and alcohol in the same period (Abel 1986). Remembering that this development took place after the rise of the women's movement in the late 1960s and 1970s, Gomberg was able to suggest that in the US at least, 'Fetal Alcohol Syndrome, by its rapid popularity, had become the locus of expression of a kind of projective rage and disapprobation towards women in North American Society, making FAS the ultimate feminine crime of fetal impairment' (Gomberg 1979).

This portrayal, which has frequently dwarfed considerations of other female drinking problems, illustrates an overriding concern with women's functions of childbearing and rearing, and suggests that anything that detracts from these is subversive and deviant, and threatens the stability of society. This recurrent theme runs through much of the popular and academic literature from ancient to modern times. Informal sanctions, if not formal ones, inhibiting female drinking and representing male attempts to proscribe and control female behaviour and reproductive capacity (Holmila 1991) are likewise not new. In practice these definitions have encompassed acceptable and non-acceptable behaviour, defining acceptable female dependency as involving a man rather than a bottle (Ettorre 1989).

Although in the past decade empirical evidence about women's drinking on a national scale in the UK has emerged (Breeze 1985; Goddard 1991) and new specialist services for women have been established (Waterson and Ettorre 1989), this distorted but powerful stereotypical view of female drinking remains. Its influence is pervasive, for even professionals continue to hold more negative views of women with alcohol problems than of men with similar problems (Smith 1992).

This stereotypical view was fully developed in much of the 1960s and 1970s clinical literature which represents women with alcohol problems as, typically, between thirty-five and forty-five years old, probably divorced or separated, prone to drinking in isolation, depressed, with a rapid onset of problems and with a poorer prognosis than a man with a similar problem (Clemmons 1985). Empirical work done at the time when much of this aetiological literature was being written demonstrates these gender differentiated clinical models in practice. The clinicians who took part in one research study were shown to expect men to be more assertive, outgoing and independent, and women to be more submissive, withdrawn and dependent (Broverman et al. 1970), so it is hardly surprising that heavy female drinking was viewed as a very unfeminine activity, showing signs of independence and flouting established norms of behaviour (Litman 1978). It is easy to see why it would be branded as more deviant than mental distress. Depression would have been seen as more passive and dependent and thus construed as appropriate feminine behaviour, showing signs of dependency on males (Carob 1987). Further evidence for the longevity of this point of view comes from a more recent study of women and men with similar stages of alcohol-related liver disease, where it was found that women had more commonly than men received psychiatric treatment in the past (Saunders *et al.* 1985). This suggests that the women were seen as more disturbed than the men, even though their physical problems were similar.

This picture of greater pathology and poorer prognosis is now seen to be inaccurate (Ross *et al.* 1988), and was also seen to be so by some contemporary commentators (e.g. Gomberg 1979). Given the stigma attached to female drinking in a situation where access to treatment is not easy, the women who do reach treatment services, and hence figure in clinical studies, may have been the most extreme 'tip of the ice-berg' (Thom 1986; Smith 1992).

All alcohol problems are subject to some stigma. British community surveys repeatedly illustrate that the term 'alcoholic' is used in a pejorative sense to refer to a person physically, psychologically and socially deteriorated, a member of a deviant minority group, or somebody who is essentially tainted (Breeze 1985). Women with alcohol problems always receive more disapprobation then men (Thom 1986; Waterson and Ettorre 1989; Mills-Hopper 1992). The connotations of sexual availability that accompany female drinking are frequently more condemned than the associations with male violence (Dzaldowski *et al.* 1988). Ettorre (1992) has drawn attention to the low self-esteem of women problem drinkers, and how they often perceive themselves in a worse light than men with similar problems.

Such double standards begin in childhood. Boys are encouraged to drink at an earlier age than girls (Lowe *et al.* 1993). In adulthood, the pub remains a largely male preserve (Hunt and Satterlee 1987). A women alone in a pub continues to denote sexual availability (Hey 1986). This lack of encouragement to view drinking as a legitimate female pursuit makes it hardly surprising that popular portrayals of women with drink problems revolve around loss of self-esteem, powerlessness, secretive drinking and a poor outlook for overcoming their problems (Harwin and Otto 1979; Denzin 1991).

Much of this stereotypical 1960s and 1970s literature repeatedly draws attention to aberrations in normal sex-role performance (Beckman 1978). Even in the 1980s the topic merited a separate chapter in a review of alcohol and the family (Leland 1982). Although 'life-events' – a topical area of research – were used to explain the onset of alcoholism in middle-aged women (Curlee 1969), these events (described as the 'empty nest syndrome') were incidents that disrupted a traditionally defined female identity rooted in husband and children (Lindbeck 1972; Corrigan 1980). This interest in sex-role performance could almost be termed a governing image, that is, a summary characterisation organised around a coherent perspective (Room 1974). Indeed sex-role disturbance has remained an important focus for some more recent clinical research on women's drinking problems (Kroft and Leichner 1987). Further evidence of this governing image is to be found in the treatment of physical damage from excess alcohol (Alcohol Concern 1990). There has been a far greater emphasis on the damage to the female rather than the male reproductive system – even though heavy consumption is linked with damage to male reproductive capacity (Waterson and Duffy 1992).

The absence of a similar organising concept based on a culturally defined sex-role in studies of male alcoholism, despite empirical evidence of equal if not greater pathology and problems, only serves to underline the greater stigmatisation and stereotyping of female drinking. It is only the ideological usefulness of these stereotypes that explains their persistence. The empirical evidence – as contemporary workers, even at the height of this approach were, and are still, only too aware, does not confirm the image of the solitary, secretive, depraved and sexually disorientated woman (Vannicelli and Nash 1984). Stereotypes exist to order ideas, to express communal values and beliefs, and to maintain social boundaries, particularly where social categories are fluid. Most people drink alcohol: to be able to sharply differentiate those with problems is reassuring (Fillmore 1985b). The central concern with female sexuality is vital, for as Curlee pointed out over twenty years ago:

Woman represents important symbols that are the bedrock of society. When angels fall, they fall disturbingly far. We would rather have them in their place, which is another way of saying that they define and make our place possible and ever more comfortable.

(Curlee 1969: 171)

Furthermore, in an ideology which sees women and motherhood as characterised by self-denying and subservient nurturing of men and off-spring alike, should the angels be pregnant or responsible for children, they have even further to fall and fall more heavily. Such ideological portrayals of motherhood inevitably conflict with stereotypical portrayals of independent and stigmatised female drinking. After all, 'Nobody likes to think that the hand that rocks the cradle might be shaky' (Curlee 1970: 247).

ACCOUNTING FOR DIFFERENT DRINKING PATTERNS: OPPORTUNITIES AND DIFFICULTIES

The following section reviews two apparently contradictory explanations for heavy drinking which commonly figure in both popular and professional literature about women's drinking. These are that drinking is either related to opportunity and possibilities, or that it is used to counteract psychological distress. The first explanation refers to situations where drinking is socially expected or appropriate and the second to difficult situations. However, neither can operate unless access to the means is possible in a material sense. Curiously, in the clinical and survey literature on women's drinking neither this link between these two perspectives nor any others are developed.

Such explanations presume that drinking behaviour is a social behaviour. Like any social behaviour once a drinking behaviour is established it will acquire an influence of its own and become part of the context which will affect future drinking behaviour. In this way past drinking patterns influence present ones, and thus an individual develops a drinking career or pathway.

Opportunities

As alcohol became more easily obtainable in the UK during the 1970s consumption rose – clearly establishing that at a societal level ease of access and increased intake are linked. The argument that follows extends this approach and looks at how access is distributed between women, particularly those of childbearing age. ||

\ It is well established that women with pre-school children are unlikely to feature among the higher consumers in any survey (Goddard and Ikin 1988; OPCS 1992). The heavier female drinkers tend to be young (under twenty-five), unmarried, without any dependent children and in regular employment (Breeze 1985; OPCS 1992).\\The explanation is that withdrawal from the labour market, with its attendant loss of income and increased domestic responsibilities combine to reduce the possibilities for drinking. In a similar vein prospective studies of drinking behaviour amongst pregnant women in this country and North America have profiled heavier drinkers as being older, of higher social status and without any dependent children (Streissguth *et al.* 1983; Heller *et al.* 1988) – in other words the women who have the opportunity to drink. In addition because they are older their earning potential has risen. Higher-income groups spend more on alcohol (Blaxter 1990).\ Community data have consistently recorded that women from professional/managerial households, who on the whole have higher incomes than other groups drink more (Breeze 1985; Goddard and Ikin 1988; Goddard 1991; Marmot *et al.* 1991; OPCS 1992).

There is now considerable evidence that women who work are likely to be heavier drinkers than those who do not (Breeze 1985; Cox *et al.* 1987; Shore 1992). Apart from an independent income, employment may also bring them into contact with drinking companions. Social contact with work friends is greater among drinkers than non-drinkers (Breeze 1985). In 1950 only 13 per cent of women with a child less than one year old were working. By the mid-1980s 7 per cent of women who had at least one pre-school child were in full-time work, and a further 20 per cent were in part-time work (Martin and Roberts 1984). By 1990 the proportion had risen to 37 per cent (OPCS 1992). The higher the level of the occupation the more common it is for women to continue working – thus reinforcing income differentials (Martin 1986).

The type of job itself may actually encourage drinking. Alcohol-related mortality rates vary widely between male occupations (Slattery *et al.* 1986). Eight factors distinguish these high-risk occupations: alcohol is likely to be freely available; there may be social pressure to drink; frequent absence from home or normal society; little close supervision; high stress and responsibility; very high or low rates of pay; colleagues may collude in heavy drinking; finally it may be that certain sorts of occupations recruit those with a predisposition to heavy drinking (Plant 1981). The evidence on women's jobs is less conclusive (Breeze 1985; Shore 1992), but as they participate more in the labour market and enter previously male-dominated jobs then it is reasonable to suppose that some of these occupational differences will emerge. Thus employment type is almost certainly an important consideration in explaining differential access to drinking.

Drinking companions acquired through employment are not the only social contacts that affect women's drinking. There is a wide variety of evidence from community surveys, clinical literature on female alcoholics, alcohol and pregnancy research and studies on the sociology of friendship to suggest that drinking norms are similar between friends and within families (Weiner *et al.* 1983; Jerome 1984; Bingol *et al.* 1987; Waterson and Murray-Lyon 1989a, 1989b). In other words, higher consuming women seem to associate with heavier drinking companions. Unfortunately, none of these studies sheds much light on the social processes which achieve these similarities.

Family cultures, and to a lesser extent friendship patterns are influenced by religious and ethnic context. Anthropologists have paid considerable interest to the regulatory effects of culture and religion on drinking in primitive societies, but there has been less interest in current European cultures (Douglas 1987). However, there is evidence that certain religious groupings drink more than others. Although alcohol is prohibited by certain religions such as Islam and Hinduism, recent empirical evidence on the influence of ethnicity suggests that some ethnic minority women do drink but on the whole they remain very light drinkers (Waterson and Murray-Lyon 1989c). This general finding that powerful norms about appropriate drinking seem to be shared between friends, family and cultural grouping is important, particularly if gender influences reinforce expectations.

Curiously (or as might be expected in the light of much of the discussion in the previous section), one factor barely figures in the literature, and that is women drinking for enjoyment. After all, the time-honoured reason for drinking is to fall under the influence, or at least to take pleasure from it. Many women like the taste of alcohol, enjoy it with meals and use it to celebrate. A study of friendship patterns amongst a group of middle-class older women by Jerome (1984) amply illustrates this point. The group met frequently to entertain each other with meals and drinking, thus providing a leisure activity and source of companionship. Breeze (1985) also found that heavier drinkers were more likely to have leisure activities which could be combined with drinking.

During the 1980s health educationalists hoped that an emphasis on 'safe' levels of consumption would restrict the social acceptability of heavy drinking. Evidence shows that the public do not see drinking as a major health concern (Blaxter 1990). The public remains confused about what levels of intake are recommended and the relative strengths of different drinks (Anderson and Wallace 1988). Following Blaxter's finding that it was only middle-class people who were concerned about the health risks of drinking, and that middle-class women are more likely to subscribe to 'official' advice on preventive health care it seems probable that if these health norms have any restrictive influence this will be most discernible amongst middle-class women. In addition, there is now a large amount of literature on lay perceptions of the causes of illness and how health can be promoted. Calnan (1987) has documented this with reference to women, showing that middle-class women tend to hold views which are congruent with those of the professionals. They are more convinced of the importance of health care advice generated from epidemiological studies and the impact of life style on health status than working-class women, who sometimes regard health education messages as a way of taking all the fun out of life (Cornwall 1984). Also, the social situation of working-class women often makes it more difficult for them to avail themselves of some of these recommended changes. Therefore, it is likely that these class differences extend to the way these groups view the use of alcohol and the recommended 'safe' levels of consumption.

To pull the threads together then, the picture is that heavier women drinkers have a high income, live in a professional/managerial household, probably work (particularly in an occupation associated with heavy drinking), move in a social milieu where heavy drinking is a shared norm, have leisure pursuits which involve drinking and are less likely to be influenced by any health norms about restricting drinking.

Difficulties

While alcohol has sedative properties, whether it really helps to reduce tension or not is debatable (De Boer *et al.* 1993). Nevertheless, it remains a common assumption that it does. In a fairly recent study, of 1,008 executives when asked of ways of reducing stress 54 per cent said they had an alcoholic drink (Harz *et al.* 1990: 11). There is some evidence that heavier women drinkers may be more likely to think that it can lift depression (Breeze 1985; Davidson and Ritson 1993). But, it is unlikely that drinking will be used to counteract all psychological difficulties or by all individuals with such difficulties. Usage will be influenced by its social and material availability and access to alternative coping strategies.

General stress, both social and psychological, is frequently cited as a cause of heavy drinking. Concepts of stress are difficult to define and even more difficult to measure (Pollock 1988). Objective indices of deprivation or difficulty can be constructed, but evaluation of the differential impact on individuals depends on context, for example the numbers of other simultaneous difficulties and the resources of the individual to meet such demands.

There is little empirical work available about whether heavier drinkers in the community report more signs of stress than lighter drinkers. Breeze (1985) found that heavier drinkers complained more that things were getting on top of them, of losing confidence, that nobody understood them, that life had no purpose, and of feeling miserable or depressed. Feeling shy in company, anxious or nervy, irritable, touchy, or worried about the future were also more commonly reported by them. This is in keeping with a report that women drink to increase self-confidence, to aid interpersonal contact, decision making or in executing some particularly demanding action (Johnson 1982). Certainly clinical reviews have frequently suggested that female alcoholics are often depressed (Corrigan 1980; Cooke and Allan 1984).

This discussion of potential sources of difficulty, both social and psychological, presumes a link between social situation – especially the availability of (material and social) support systems – and psychological unease.

North American studies of pregnant women carried out in deprived inner-city areas found that the heaviest drinkers had multiple social problems (Weiner *et al.* 1983; Stephens 1985). One

British study has also indicated a small pocket of heavy drinkers with social difficulties (Heller *et al.* 1988), and several British studies have reported that smoking, which has been described as a sign of deprivation (Oakley 1989) was associated with drinking (Sulaiman *et al.* 1988; Waterson and Murray Lyon 1989a; 1989b).

Material support gives security. If finances are sufficient other supports such as domestic help, child care and transport can be purchased. For despite an apparent trend towards greater father participation in child care (Lewis and O'Brien 1987) women still take primary responsibility for housework and child care even if working (Brannen and Moss 1991). Those who can afford to pay for help have a material buffer against stress arising from these demands. Single mothers living on a low income with no domestic help or practical supports are likely to experience the greatest difficulties.

The social network of family and close friends is not only a source of support but strengthens an individual's sense of identity (Oakley and Rajan 1991; O'Connor 1991; Franks 1992). Furthermore, it can guard against psychological difficulties by acting as a defence in the face of sudden difficulties (Brown and Harris 1989). The quality of this support is important. Being sure of help in a crisis and 'being there' may be just as important as frequent contact (Brannen and Moss 1988). Those with limited social networks and who lack a confidant are likely to experience the greatest difficulties and be most vulnerable in the face of sudden changes such as the transition to motherhood. There is now increasing evidence to show that these two types of support interact. In a study of women's confidantes outside marriage, O'Connor (1991) found that those who experienced marital and financial insecurity were also least likely to have a confidante. Oakley and Rajan (1990) compared social support amongst middle-class and working-class mothers with young children. They found that the working-class mothers were less involved with their families and were more socially isolated in terms of friends. They were also less likely to receive any male domestic support – practical or emotional.

Existing data connecting these factors with drinking are sparse. Breeze (1985) found that the heaviest drinkers were least likely to have a confidante. Physical difficulties, in particular those relating to gynaecological or obstetric concerns, have featured in the clinical literature on women's drinking problems (Wilsnack

1985). Early motherhood – when women are faced with a demanding baby, involving increased practical and emotional demands, as well as having to continue to meet the dependency needs of her partner – is likely to test these supports.

For those women who are combining work with child care, employment demands can lead to role strain and work over-load, with its attendant time pressures and fatigue. Women's employment is still considered something to be accommodated to domestic requirements (Brannen and Moss 1991). Indeed, female alcoholics have often recorded their guilt at not being a 'proper' mother who is at home with the children (Volicer *et al.* 1981). Women with higher-status occupations are less inclined to subscribe to the traditional view that 'a woman's place is in the home' (Brannen and Moss 1991), and often derive intrinsic rewards from their work. They are more likely to be able to purchase domestic help and are also more likely to have more flexible jobs and be able to control their working arrange-ments more. Women with lower-status jobs do not have the same advantages. If they also hold traditional views about women with children working and are only working for financial reasons then they may well find work less rewarding (Martin 1986).

The contrast between romantic conceptualisations of pregnancy and motherhood that characterise popular literature and media portrayals and the reality are enormous. Those women who give up employment lose status, income and become more isolated (Oakley 1974, 1980). Many women find that their experience of motherhood does not measure up to their expectations. In the face of this dissonance they feel inadequate. This is another way of looking at the sex-role conflict, which as noted earlier, has been such a dominant preoccupation in the literature. Some of these studies used fairly simplistic psychological tests to try to demon-strate conflict between unconscious femininity and conscious masculinity or vice versa (Leland 1982). The direction of such conflicts still remains unclear (Kroft and Leichner 1987), but what is important is that these studies presume that drinking dimin-ishes this sense of dissonance which frequently emanates from the gap between experience and hopes and desires. There is some evidence that amongst housewives with identified alcohol problems, the severity of the problem may be related to the degree of dissatisfaction with their role (Farid *et al.* 1989). If this discrepancy and disappointment is marked then drinking to dispel feelings of dissatisfaction seems plausible.

There is now a considerable body of literature demonstrating that 'life-events', or significant changes in the on-going life pattern of an individual – such as a role transformation, a marked change in health, domestic or social status or environment – are associated with a wide range of physical and psychological difficulties (Brown and Harris 1989). However, this body of research is riddled with methodological difficulties. The consensus is that they may be important in explaining the onset of alcohol problems but data on women are few (Gorman and Peters 1990). In one sample of 132 women, heavy drinking was not linked with 'life-events', but was with depression (Cooke and Allan 1984). In another study, Thom (1986) found that 50 per cent of her sample of women in treatment for alcohol problems reported that significant 'life-events' had precipitated their heavy drinking. One criticism of this study is that heavy female drinking is highly stigmatised and some women may try to reduce their sense of stigma by ascribing their problems to a specific cause. This is particularly likely as it is often a 'life-event' that precipitates them into treatment (Thom 1986).

Breeze (1985) found that the very heavy drinkers in her community survey were slightly more likely than the rest of the sample to have recently separated, changed partners or been worried about a partner. This is in keeping with many other studies which have drawn attention to higher consumption levels amongst divorced and separated women (Heller *et al.* 1988; OPCS 1992; Goddard 1991). On the other hand Breeze also found that illnesses, accidents, losing a job, moving to a new area, or bereavement were not more common amongst heavy drinkers. It seems that it was occurrences where women's dependency on their partners was threatened that were most significant. In addition, it is noticeable that all the 'life-events' mentioned in the Thom study, which included divorce, separation, diagnosis of infertility and the birth of a handicapped child, related to their ability to perform a traditional female role. The only exception was bereavement. Those events which threaten the self-esteem associated with female role performance do appear to be highly significant.

To summarise then, the picture which emerges from the literature is that heavy drinkers show more signs of psychological distress, are less well materially and socially supported, have more difficulties with employment, suffer from more physical troubles, may be less satisfied with their experience of motherhood, and have been more exposed to 'life-events', particularly those which threaten a sense of self-esteem, than lighter drinkers. ¡\

SIXTY WOMEN'S EXPERIENCES

The final part of this chapter takes some of these themes, and recounts how important they were to a group of women whose drinking patterns had been charted over a period of approximately three years. These women all had at least one small child under three years old and had been enrolled into a prospective study looking at drinking patterns during pregnancy and early mother-hood. None of them were identified problem drinkers, but some were heavier drinkers than others (Waterson 1992).

The sixty were selected from the last 250 women enrolled into a large epidemiological study sample drawn from the ante-natal clinic of a London teaching hospital. After excluding women who lived outside the catchment area of Greater London and those who moved away during the follow up time a group of 222 women were left. The 222 were divided into those drawn from a professional/managerial background (defined by social class of head of household and associated with higher income, greater access to material supports, higher educational and housing status) and others (who were less advantaged in terms of income, education, domestic support and education). They were further sub-divided according to their drinking level when they first enrolled at the ante-natal clinic some years before. These women were all pregnant at the time and their consumption levels had dropped off. So, those drinking more than ten units of alcohol a week or more were defined as the heavier drinkers and those drinking less than that the lighter drinkers. Ten units per week is the lowest level at which alcohol consumption has been demonstrated to affect pregnancy outcome in terms of indicators such as a reduced birth weight. Women need to be drinking considerably more (35+ units a week) to run any significant risk of producing a child with Fetal Alcohol Syndrome, which is a permanent condition affecting both phys-ical and mental development. None of these women were drinking at such levels.

The women were divided into four groups:

- professional/managerial heavier drinkers (PMH);
- professional/managerial lighter drinkers (PML);
- other heavier drinkers (OH);
- other lighter drinkers (OL).

The distribution of the 222 women between the four groups is shown in Table 7.1. The key point is that professional women were almost twice as likely to be heavier drinkers than women in any of the other groups.

Fifteen women from each group were interviewed about their experiences over the past three or four years. The study was presented as a general one rather than one concentrating specifically on drinking. Consequently it was not possible to pursue some questions to their logical conclusions. Secondly the lack of research looking at drinking amongst women without identified problems in any depth made a 'broad brush' approach inevitable.

The most obvious finding was that pregnancy did affect drinking habits. They almost all cut down their drinking, but the heavier drinkers remained the heavier drinkers throughout the whole time period. These differences in drinking patterns revealed a major division between higher and lower consumers, which were maintained throughout pregnancy and early motherhood. This was because at anyone time a woman's drinking pattern was the result of a negotiated 'career', involving an interaction between past drinking practices and current structural and cultural influences.

The two themes of opportunity and drinking and difficulties and drinking were clearly recognisable and frequently intermingled.

Table 7.1 Women's drinking levels by social class

	SOCIAL CLASS		
	Professional/ managerial (PM) (%)	Other (O) (%)	All (%)
Drinking level			
Heavier (H)	32	18	25
Lighter (L)	68	82	75
Base (=100%)	114	108	222

Social reasons, relating to social expectations and practices as well as personal preferences were the most important reasons for drinking at all levels of consumption. It was only the higher consumers who mentioned reasons relating to difficulties, and even then they hastily cited social reasons as well.

Turning to the women's perceptions and their objective experiences these themes can be elaborated. Opportunity and access factors were important and included measures of material situation, social status and employment and social contacts, as well as social norms. Difficulties fell into two main types: objective measures of social and material disadvantage, and those arising from changing circumstances. Some of these were objective difficulties such as physical problems or little social contact. Others were subjective, for example expressed dissatisfaction. A third set of factors – social norms about drinking and personal attitudes towards it – were independent of either of these two main themes.

Let us look at these four groups and their different drinking pathways in more detail. It was apparent that the heavier drinkers (H) were more inclined to enjoy drinking, valued socialising and used alcohol to help them relax. Such attitudes were shared by friends and family. Not surprisingly, they were disinclined to heed any health education warnings about 'safe' levels of consumption that might interfere with this. These attitudes preceded motherhood and remained largely unaffected by it. If these H drinkers found drinking both relaxing and enjoyable, then using it to ameliorate minor psychological unease would seem to be not only understandable but probable.

However, not all H drinkers had equal opportunities to drink. It was obvious that the professional/managerial (PM) women had enhanced opportunities both before and during motherhood. They came from wealthier households, and were more able to purchase both alcohol and leisure in which to drink it. For them, unlike the other women (O) there were no sanctions against drinking at home. By contrast, the O women were disadvantaged. They were worse off, more likely to have housing problems, more likely to be without independent transport and to receive less practical help. These disadvantages discouraged H drinking. As Table 7.1 shows, H drinking was unusual among the O women. In motherhood the PM women were more likely to have continued working and to have maintained a source of independent disposable income as well as contact with work-based drinking companions and friends. More O women gave up work after giving birth so that their households were more often reliant on one income, thus widening the existing differentials. This disadvantage not only affected their opportunity to drink but also their quality of life. It also made them more vulnerable to the difficulties which arose in motherhood.

These positions are highlighted when the PMH and OH drinkers are compared. In addition to the difficulties outlined above, the OH group were particularly vulnerable to housing problems. On the other hand, the PMH group had even more enhanced material status than the PML group. Alcohol was constantly available at home. Drinking alone was not taboo. Their partners, who often worked in 'alcohol risk' occupations, were high consumers and supportive of their drinking. They had more frequent contact with their family members which often involved drinking. However, in comparison with their lighter-drinking peers (L) both groups of H drinkers had additional possibilities of access to alcohol. They were slightly better off and were more likely to have worked or be working in an occupation associated with high alcohol usage.

Both PM and O women had specific difficulties. PM women complained of time pressures and were dissatisfied with the amount of social contact they were able to sustain. They were also exposed to more deeply upsetting 'life-events', though the O women experienced more 'life-events' altogether. The O women had less contact with women with young children, had more physically and psychologically troublesome pregnancies, were more often disappointed with the reality of giving birth, prone to depressed mood or depression post-natally, more disappointed with the realities of child care and their current situation. More of them were distinguished as being in need of psychiatric assessment at interview.

Both groups of H drinkers experienced some of these problems more severely. In comparison with their L peers, regardless of the amount of social contact they had they were more discontented about it. They found their initial experiences of child care particularly disappointing. In addition, they had more psychological problems and were more inclined to have physical problems at all stages.

For each H group certain difficulties were felt more keenly. Of all the groups the OH drinkers were most disappointed with the experience of pregnancy, and experienced both more frequent, and more upsetting 'life-events' than their OL peers. The PMH group were especially unhappy with not seeing their friends enough and with having to cope with time pressures.

The opportunity factors, encouraging of drinking and the disadvantages and difficulties encountered by the sixty women which might have stimulated them to use drink as a coping strategy were then grouped together under four heads: attitudes towards drinking; opportunity or access factors; factors of disadvantage (social); and individual difficulties or problems. Obviously some of these factors are inter-linked and measurement was crude. Nevertheless, although they were not necessarily equally influential in promoting drinking, looking at these indications of the cumulative experience of each group relative to the others is useful. To do this each group was given a score of one for each factor that it experienced. A score for each of the four categories of factors was calculated for each group (see Table 7.2).

For example, five attitudes likely to promote drinking were distinguished. Both groups of H drinkers displayed all five and thus scored five each – the L groups scoring 0. Similarly, the PM groups had four enhanced opportunity factors in common. However, the PMH group experienced three extra opportunity factors. In addition, they and the OH group enjoyed two additional access factors. Thus, the PMH group scored nine for opportunity/access factors, the PML group four, the OH group two and the OL group nil.

When all four categories of factors are looked at cumulatively (Table 7.2) it is obvious that both H groups were considerably

Table 7.2   The distribution of four types of factors associated with drinking levels

	GROUP				
	PML	PMH	OH	OL	Total
Type of factor					
Attitudes	0	5	5	0	10
Opportunity/access	4	9	2	0	15
Disadvantage	0	0	5	4	9
Difficulties	3	9	11	5	28
Totals	7	23	23	9	62

more encouraged to drink than either L group. Interestingly, the total scores of both H groups were identical and there was little difference between the scores of the two L groups.

Both groups of H drinkers had an equal number of positive attitudes towards drinking. The PM women clearly had considerably more opportunity and access to drink. The combined score for opportunity and access for the two PM groups is thirteen, but only two for the combined two O groups. The O groups were obviously much more disadvantaged than the PM women. They also experienced more difficulties (sixteen) as compared with the PM women (twelve).

Looking at these distributions it could be imagined that if any group would be likely to drink as a means of coping with difficulties it would be the OH group. They were the most disadvantaged and experienced the greatest number of difficulties of any group. Similarly, if any group was likely to drink because they were encouraged by opportunity it would be the PMH group. Women in the PMH group were not without their problems, but the impact of some difficulties would be buffered by their social advantage.

None the less, the two H groups experienced different sorts of problems and especially pinpointed certain difficulties pertaining to female role performance. These included separating from a partner and a less than ideal performance as a mother due to post-natal depression. In this context, physically difficult pregnancies, psychological troubles and dissatisfaction and disappointment with pregnancy, giving birth or motherhood could also be thought of as indications of a less than ideal maternal performance. All groups apart from the PML group experienced some of these types of difficulties, but it was the OH group who felt more of them and felt them most keenly. They held the most traditional views about motherhood but their material constraints made it difficult for them to achieve such roles.

The PMH women experienced fewer such role-performance difficulties. Their particular complaints seemed to centre around the highly organised, complex and pressured lives they led. It was this group that mentioned regular daily drinking and who were comfortable drinking alone. In this situation, it is easy to imagine that in circumstances which could easily get out of control they used drink to maintain equilibrium, to restore a sense of balance and consequently their self-esteem. For the OH group it is more credible that they seized their more limited opportunities in early motherhood for drinking more as a means of 'drowning their sorrows.' For both groups such drinking could be seen as constructive if it helped them to cope better at other times.

This last point brings us back full circle to the argument described earlier in this chapter, that concepts of faulty female sex-role performance can be seen as a central theme in the past and current literature about drinking in pregnancy and motherhood. This analysis suggests that there may be some truth in that focus, but that it needs redefining in a social context. Rather than such problems being due to individual irresponsibility, ignorance or psychological conflict they are quite clearly structurally and culturally shaped, and reflect other inequalities.

This issue should not be laboured, however, because it is also equally obvious that factors of opportunity are a much more powerful explanation of high consumption than using alcohol as a coping mechanism. Furthermore, only those women with positive attitudes towards drinking were likely to avail themselves of what opportunities they had to drink, or to use it as a coping device.

This is not to suggest that all heavier drinkers become problem drinkers, but these empirical data do illustrate the circumstances in which different groups of women might drift into difficulties. Primary care workers need to be aware of these different scenarios both in terms of prevention and identification of problems – but also as aids to more therapeutic work at both individual and social levels.

REFERENCES

Abel, E. L. (1984) *Fetal Alcohol Syndrome and Fetal Alcohol Effects*, London: Plenum Press.

Abel, E. (1986) 'Publication trends for alcohol, tobacco, and narcotics in MEDLARS', *Annals New York Academy of Science*, 477: 103–4.

Alcohol Concern (1990) *Warning: Alcohol Can Damage Your Health*, London: Alcohol Concern.

Anderson, P. and Wallace, P. (1988) 'Safe limits of drinking: patients views', *British Medical Journal*, 296: 1787.

Bailey, S. (1990) 'Women with alcohol problems: a psycho-social perspective', *Drug and Alcohol Review*, 9: 143–53

Beckman, L. J. (1978) 'Sex-role conflict in alcoholic women: myth or reality', *Journal of Abnormal Psychology*, 87: 408–17.

Beory, M. D. and Merry, J. (1986) 'The rise in alcoholism in women of fertile age', *British Journal of Addiction*, 81: 142.

Berridge, V. and Edwards, G. (1981) *Opium and the People: Opiate Use in Nineteenth Century England*, London: Allen Lane.

Bingol, N., Schuster, C., Fuchs, M., Aosub, S., Turner, G., Stone, R. K. and Gromisch, D. S. (1987) 'The influence of socioeconomic factors on the occurrence of Fetal Alcohol Syndrome', *Advances in Alcohol and Substance Abuse*, 6: 105–18.

Blaxter, M. (1990) *Health and Lifestyles*, London: Tavistock Routledge.

Blume, S. (1991) 'Sexuality and stigma: the alcoholic women', *Alcohol Health and Research World*, 15: 139–46.

Booth, C. (ed.) (1902) *Life and Labour of the People of London: Notes on Social Influences and Conclusion*, London: Macmillan.

Brannen, J. and Moss, P. (1988) *New Mothers at Work*, London: Unwin Hyman.

Brannen, J. and Moss, P. (1991) *Managing Mothers: Dual Earner Households after Maternity Leave*, London: Unwin Hyman.

Breeze, E. (1985) *Women and Drinking*, London: HMSO.

Broverman, I. K., Broverman, D. M., Clarkson, F. E., Rosenkrantz, P. S. and Vogel, S. R. (1970) 'Sex-role stereotypes and clinical judgements of mental health', *Journal of Consulting and Clinical Psychology*, 34: 1–7.

Brown, G. and Harris, T. (1989) *Life Events and Illness: a Reference Book for the Caring Professions*, London: Routledge.

Calnan, M. (1987) *Health and Illness: the Lay Perspective*, London: Tavistock.

Carob, A. (1987) *Working with Depressed Women*, Aldershot: Gower.

Cherpital, C. J. (1994) 'Alcohol and casualties: a comparison of emergency room and coroner data', *Alcohol and Alcoholism*, 29: 211–18.

Clemmons, P. (1985) 'Reflections of social thought in research on women and alcoholism', *Journal of Drug Issues*, 15: 73–80.

Cooke, D. J. and Allan, C. A. (1984) 'Stressful life events and alcohol abuse in women: a general population study', *British Journal of Addiction*, 79: 425–31.

Cornwall, J. (1984) *Hard-earned Lives: Accounts of Health and Illness from East London*, London: Tavistock.

Corrigan, E. M. (1980) *Alcoholic Women in Treatment*, New York: Oxford University Press.

Coupe, J. (1992) 'Why women need their own services', in Glass, I. (ed.) *The International Handbook of Addictive Behaviour*, Tavistock/ Routledge, London.

Cox, B. D., Blaxter, M. and Buckle, A. (1987) *Health and Lifestyle Survey: Preliminary Report*, Cambridge: Health Promotion Trust.

Curlee, J. (1969) 'Alcoholism and the empty nest', *Bulletin of the Menninger Clinic*, 33: 165–71.

Curlee, J. (1970) 'A comparison of male and female patients at an alcoholism treatment centre', *Journal of Psychology*, 74; 239–47.

Davidson, K., Ritson, E. B., (1993) 'The relationship between alcohol dependence and depression', *Alcohol and Alcoholism*, 28: 147–55.

DAWN (1988) *Black Women and Dependency: a Report on Drug and Alcohol Use*, London: DAWN.

DAWN (1994) *Survey of Facilities for Women Using Drugs (Including Alcohol) in London*, London: DAWN.

De Boer, N. C., Schippers, G. M., Van Der Staak, C. P. F. (1993) 'Alcohol and social anxiety in women and men: pharmacological and expectancy effects', *Addictive Behaviors*, 18: 117–26.

Department of Health and Royal College of General Practitioners (1992) *Women and Alcohol*, London HMSO.

Denzin, N. K. (1991) *Hollywood by Shot: Alcoholism in the American Cinema*, New York: Aldine De Gruyter.

Douglas, M. (1987) *Constructive Drinking*, Cambridge: Cambridge University Press.

Dzaldowski, A., Heather, N. and Crawford, J. (1988) 'Perceptions of drinkers and abstainers in a sample of Scottish adults', *Alcohol and Alcoholism*, 23: 7–16.

Ettorre, B. (1989) 'Women and substance use/abuse: towards a feminist perspective', *Women's Studies International Forum*, 12: 593–602.

Ettorre, E., (1992) *Women and Substance Use*, Macmillan, London.

Farid, B., Elsherbini, M., Ogden, M., Lucas, G. and Williams, R. (1989) 'Alcoholic housewives and role satisfaction', *Alcohol and Alcoholism*, 24: 331–37.

Ferrence, R. G. (1980) 'Sex differences in the prevalence of problem drinking', in Kalant, O. (ed.) *Alcohol and Drug Problems in Women*, New York: Plenum Press.

Fillmore, K. (1985a) 'The social victims of drinking', *British Journal of Addiction*, 80: 307–14.

Fillmore, K. M. (1985b) '"When angels fall": Women's drinking as cultural preoccupation and as reality', in S. C., Wilsnack and L. J. Beckman (eds) *Alcohol Problems in Women: Antecedents, Consequences, and Intervention*, New York: Guilford Press.

Franks, P. (1992) 'Social relationships and health: the relative roles of family functioning and social support', *Social Science and Medicine*, 34: 779–88.

Goddard, E. (1991) *Drinking in England and Wales in the Late 1980s*, London: HMSO.

Goddard, E. and Ikin, C. (1988) *Drinking in England and Wales in 1987*, London: HMSO.

Gomberg, E. S. (1979) 'Drinking patterns of women alcoholics', in V. Burtle (ed.) *Women Who Drink*, Springfield, IL: Thomas Books.

Gomberg, E. S. (1993) 'Alcohol, women and the expression of aggression', *Journal of Studies on Alcohol*, Supplement 11: 89–95.

Gorman, D. M. and Peters, T. J. (1990) 'Types of life events and the onset of alcohol dependence', *British Journal of Addiction*, 85: 71–9.

Gutzke, D. (1984) '"The cry of the children"': the Edwardian medical campaign against maternal drinking', *British Journal of Addiction*, 79: 71–84.

Harwin, J. and Otto, S. (1979) 'Women, alcohol and the screen', in J. Cook and M. Lewington (eds) *Images of Alcoholism*, London: British Film Institute/Alcohol Education Centre.

Harz, C., Plant, M. A. and Watts, M. (1990) *Alcohol and Health: a Handbook for Nurses, Midwives, and Health Visitors*, London: Medical Council on Alcoholism.

Heller, J., Anderson, H. R., Bland, J. M., Brooke, O. G., Peacock, J. L. and Stewart, C. M. (1988) 'Alcohol in pregnancy: patterns and association with the socioeconomic, psychological and behavioural factors', *British Journal of Addiction*, 83: 541–51.

Hey, V. (1986) *Patriarchy and Pub Culture*, London: Tavistock.

Holmila, M. (1991) 'Social control experienced by heavily drinking women', *Contemporary Drug Problems*, 2: 547–71.

Hunt, G. (1988) 'Wretched, hatless and misclad: women and the inebriate reformatories from 1900–1913', *British Journal of Sociology*, 40; 245–70.

Hunt, G. and Satterlee, S. (1987) 'Darts, drink and the pub: the culture of female drinking', *Sociological Review*, 3: 575–601.

Jerome, D. (1984) 'Good company: The sociological implications of friendship', *Sociological Review*, 32: 696–718.

Johnson, N. B. (1982) 'Sex differences, Women's roles and alcohol use: preliminary national data, *Journal of Social Issues*, 38: 93–116.

Kalant, O. J. (ed.) (1980) *Alcohol and Drug Problems in Women*, Advances in Alcohol and Drug Problems, New York: Plenum.

Kroft, C. and Leichner, P. (1987) 'Sex-role conflicts in alcoholic women', *International Journal of Addictions*, 22: 685–693.

Leland, J. (1982) 'Sex roles, family organisation and alcohol abuse', in J. Orford and J. Harwin, (eds) *Alcohol and the Family*, London: Croom Helm.

Lewis, J. (1980) *The Politics of Motherhood: Child and Maternal Welfare in England 1900–1939*, London: Croom Helm.

Lewis, J. (1986) 'Anxieties about the family and the relationships between parents, children and the state in twentieth century England', in M. Richards and P. Light (eds) *Children of Social Worlds*, Cambridge: Polity Press.

Lewis, J. (1991) *Women and Social Action in Victorian and Edwardian England*, London: Edward Elgar.

Lewis, C. and O'Brien, M. (1987) *Reassessing Fatherhood*, London: Sage Publications.

Lindbeck, V. L. (1972) 'The woman alcoholic: a review of the literature', *International Journal of the Addictions*, 7: 567–80.

Lisansky, E. (1957) 'Alcoholism in women: social and psychological concomitants', *Quarterly Journal of Studies on Alcohol*, 18: 588–623.

Litman, G. (1978) 'Clinical aspects of sex role stereotyping', in J. Chetwyn and O. Hartnett (eds) *The Sex Role System*, London: Routledge & Kegan Paul.

Lowe, G., Foxcroft, D. and Sibley, D. (1993) *Adolescent Drinking and Family Life*, London: Harwood Academic Press.

Marmot, M. G., Davey-Smith, G., Stansfield, S., Patel, C., North, F., Head, J., White, I., Brunner, E. and Feeney, A. (1991) 'Health inequalities among British civil servants: the Whitehall II study', *British Medical Journal*, 337: 1387–93.

Martin, J. and Roberts, C. (1984) *Women and Employment*, London: HMSO.

Martin, J. (1986) 'Returning to work after childbearing; evidence from the women and employment survey', *Population Trends*, 43: 23–30.

McDonald, M. (1994) *Gender, Drink and Drugs*, Berg: Oxford.

Mills-Hopper (1992) *Alcohol Concern: Women and Alcohol – a Research Based Evaluation*, London: Mills-Hopper Associates for Alcohol Concern.

McDowell, L. (1989) 'Gender Divisions', in C. Hamnett, L. McDowell and P. Sarre (eds) *Restructuring Britain: The Changing Social Structure*, London: Sage.

Oakley, A. (1974) The *Sociology of Housework*, Oxford: Martin Robertson.

Oakley, A. (1980) *Women Confined*, Oxford: Martin Robertson.

Oakley, A. (1989) 'Smoking in pregnancy: smokecreen or risk factor? Towards a materialistic analysis', *Sociology of Health and Illness*, 11: 311–35.

Oakley, A. and Rajan, L. (1991) 'Social class and social support: the same or different?', *Sociology*, 25: 31–60.

O'Connor, P. (1991) 'Women's confidants outside marriage: shared or competing sources of intimacy', *Sociology*, 25: 241–54.

(OPCS) Office of Population Censuses and Surveys (1992) *General Household Survey 1990*, London: HMSO.

Plant, M. P. (1981) 'Risk factors in employment', in B. D. Hore and M. P. Plant (eds) *Alcohol Problems in Employment*, London: Croom Helm.

Plant, M. (1990) *Women and Alcohol: a Review of International Literature on the Use of Alcohol by Females*, Geneva: World Health Organisation Publications.

Pollock, K. (1988) 'On the nature of social status: production of a modern mythology', *Social Science and Medicine*, 26: 381–92.

Room, R. (1974) 'Governing images and the prevention of alcohol problems', *Preventive Medicine*, 3: 11–23.

Ross, H. E., Glaser, F. B. and Stiansy, S. (1988) 'Sex differences in the prevalence of psychiatric disorders in patients with alcohol and drug problems', *British Journal of Addiction*, 83: 1179–92.

Rowbotham, S. (1990) *The Past is Before Us: Feminism in Action Since the 1960s*, London: Penguin.

Royal College of General Practitioners (1986) *Alcohol – a Balanced View*, London: Royal College of General Practitioners.

Saunders, J. H., Wodak, A. D. and Williams, R. (1985) 'Past experience of advice and treatment for drinking problems of patients with alcoholic liver disease', *British Journal of Addiction*, 80: 51–6.

Shaw, S. (1980) 'The causes of increasing drinking problems amongst women', in Camberwell Council on Alcoholism (ed.) *Women and Alcohol*, London: Tavistock.

Shore, E. R. (1992) 'Drinking patterns and problems among women in paid employment', *Alcohol Health and Research World*, 16: 160–4.

Slattery, M., Alderson, M. R.and Bryant J. E. (1986) 'Occupational risks of alcoholism', *International Journal of Addictions*, 21: 929–36.

Smith, L. (1992) 'Help-seeking in alcohol-dependent females', *Alcohol and Alcoholism*, 27: 1, 3–9.

Stephens, C. J. (1985) 'Perception of pregnancy and social support as predictors of alcohol consumption during pregnancy', *Alcoholism:*

Clinical and Experimental Research, 9: 344–48.

Streissguth, A. P., Darby, B. L., Barr, H. M., Smith, J. R. and Martin, D. C. (1983) 'Comparison of drinking and smoking patterns during pregnancy over a six year interval', *American Journal of Obstetrics and Gynaecology*, 145: 716–24.

Sulaiman, N., Florey, C. du V. and Taylor, D. (1988) 'Alcohol consumption in Dundee primagravidas and its effects on outcome of pregnancy', *British Medical Journal*, 296: 1500–3.

Sullivan, W. C. (1899) 'A note on the influence of maternal inebriety on the offspring', *Journal of Mental Science*, 45: 489–503.

Thom, B. (1986) 'Sex differences in help-seeking for alcohol problems I: The barriers to help-seeking', *British Journal of Addiction*, 81: 777–88.

Vannicelli, M. and Nash, L. (1984) 'Effect of sex bias on women's studies on alcoholism', *Alcoholism: Clinical and Experimental Research*, 8: 334–36.

Vogt, I. (1984) 'Defining alcohol problems as a repressive mechanism: Its formative phase in Imperial Germany and its strength today', *International Journal of Addictions*, 19: 551–69.

Volicer, B. J., Cahil, M. H. and Smith, J. L. (1981) 'Sex differences in correlates of problem drinking among employed males and females', *Drug and Alcohol Dependence*, 8: 175–87.

Waterson, J. (1992) 'Women and alcohol: the social context of changing patterns of use in pregnancy and early motherhood', unpublished PhD thesis, London School of Economics, University of London.

Waterson, J. and Duffy, J. C., (1992) 'Alcohol damage to the foetus and reproductive system', in Duffy, J. C. (ed.) *Health Risks Associated with Alcohol Consumption*, Edinburgh: Edinburgh University Press.

Waterson, J. and Ettorre, B. (1989) 'Providing services for women with difficulties with alcohol or other drugs: the current UK situation as seen by women practitioners, researchers and policy makers in the field', *Drug and Alcohol Dependence*, 24: 119–25.

Waterson, E. J. and Murray-Lyon, I. M. (1989a) 'Drinking and smoking patterns amongst women attending an ante natal clinic I: before pregnancy', *Alcohol and Alcoholism*, 24: 153–62.

Waterson, E. J. and Murray-Lyon, I. M. (1989b) 'Drinking and smoking patterns amongst women attending an ante natal clinic II: during pregnancy', *Alcohol and Alcoholism*, 24: 163–73.

Waterson, E. J. and Murray-Lyon, I. M. (1989c) 'Alcohol, smoking and pregnancy: some observations on ethnic minorities in the United Kingdom', *British Journal of Addiction*, 84: 323–25.

Weiner, L., Rosett, H. L., Edelin, K. C. Alpert, J. and Zuckerman, B. (1983) 'Alcohol consumption by pregnant women', *Obstetrics and Gynaecology*, 61: 6–12.

Wilsnack, S. C. (1985) 'Drinking, sexuality and sexual dysfunction in women', in S. C. Wilsnack and L. J. Beckman (eds) *Alcohol Problems in Women: Antecedents, Consequences and Intervention*, New York: Guilford Press.

(WHO) World Health Organisation (1992) *Women and Substance Abuse 1992 Interim Report*, Geneva: World Health Organization.

Chapter 8

Services for women: the way forward

Betsy Thom and Anna Green

INTRODUCTION

As Chapter 7 established, women drink less alcohol than men, experience fewer alcohol-related harms, and are less likely to be involved in alcohol-related crime or accidents as a result of their own drinking. Such gender differences in the use and problem use of alcohol persist across countries, cultures and time periods (Roman 1988; Plant 1990; Goddard 1991; WHO 1992). In spite of this, over the last twenty years women have been targeted as a neglected group 'lost' to treatment, and increasingly, as a group at 'high risk' from alcohol consumption (Plant 1990a; WHO 1992).

To understand why women's drinking has gained a higher profile than at any other time this century, and why the provision of specialist services for women is a matter of debate, it is necessary to consider the social and ideological roots of present wisdom regarding women's drinking. With this in mind, we start this chapter with an overview of the forces which have shaped current discussion on the extent and nature of service provision for women. We then examine the research evidence for the influence of gender on treatment entry and treatment outcome. Finally, we consider the question of the need for specialist services for women and for gender-sensitive treatment approaches.

Gender roles and alcohol use

Women's use of alcoholic beverages has always been subject to greater social control and restriction than that of men; equally, women's misuse of alcohol has attracted greater condemnation, greater punishment and greater shame (Litman 1975). The emphasis placed in most cultures on women's gender-based roles – their duties as wives, mothers, carers and, more broadly, as the 'moral guardians' of society – provides the common thread in attitudes running through Biblical pronouncements on foetal harm (Judges 13, 2–7), through the concerns of the Roman Empire to protect patrimonial rights (Jellinek 1976), or through eugenic arguments in early twentieth century England that women's drinking was a prominent factor in the 'degeneration of the race' (Kelynack 1902).

In the post-1950s resurgence of interest in women's drinking, the phrase 'alcoholism represents the ransom woman pays for her emancipation' conveys a similarly gloomy forecast for women in an era of change in traditional gender roles (Massot *et al.* 1956). In short, women's misuse of alcohol – however 'misuse' is defined in a society – is generally seen as particularly threatening to the social order. As a result, where formal laws and regulations do not differentiate between male and female rights to use alcohol, informal controls and sanctions can often impose powerful restraints on women's alcohol consumption, on their drinking behaviour, and on the actions they take when their drinking becomes problematic (see Holmila 1991).

For the greater part of this century women's drinking has received little attention. The introduction of legislation to curb alcohol consumption at the turn of the century, the economic depression of the 1930s and restrictions on the availability of alcohol in the years during and after the Second World War, were important factors in keeping *per capita* consumption low in the UK (see Williams and Brake 1980).

According to the Ministry of Health, in the 1950s the UK had no alcohol problem (see Chapter 10). The dominant view – that there was a minority of individuals who suffered from the disease of 'alcoholism' – separated the most severely afflicted drinkers from those with less visible or extreme drinking problems, and deflected attention away from the drinking habits of the population as a whole. By the early 1960s the Ministry of Health, succumbing to pressure to provide an official treatment response to the problem of 'alcoholism', had recommended the establishment of specialist alcohol treatment units in each health authority region (see Thom and Berridge 1995).

During this period, there were women among the visible minority of 'alcoholics' but they were few in number, and although some services attempted to address their needs, pronouncements regarding treatment approaches were derived largely from a consideration of male drinkers (Glatt 1982: 165). Later critics of the services and treatment approaches available to women in the 1960s and 1970s pointed out that the field abounded in myths concerning the woman drinker – as untypical of her sex, as problematic to treat and as having a poorer prognosis than her male counterpart (Litman 1975; Annis and Liban 1980; Camberwell Council on Alcoholism 1980; Glatt 1982).

It may well be that lack of public and professional awareness of women's drinking, the stigma surrounding women's alcoholism and the inadequate nature of available treatment responses brought only the most disturbed and severely damaged women to the notice of treatment agencies (Glatt 1982). Undoubtedly, the impressions and clinical experience of those women who sought treatment underpinned the prevailing view of women drinkers both in the UK and abroad: few research studies included enough women to examine the truth or otherwise of clinical observation and anecdote (Vannicelli and Nash 1984). Until the survey by Wilson in 1980, followed by the survey by Breeze in the early 1980s (Breeze 1985), there was no national picture of women's alcohol consumption in the UK. However, in the ten years between 1970 and 1980, the alcohol field changed profoundly with far-reaching consequences for responses to women's alcohol consumption and problem drinking.

By 1980, the emphasis was no longer firmly fixed on 'alcoholism' and the 'alcoholic'. A new 'public health' approach to alcohol had swung attention away from the disease concept and those most severely affected by drinking, towards a concern with the drinking patterns and habits of the population as a whole (Baggott 1990). This broader perspective of the alcohol problem, drew attention to the consumption habits of people who were not 'alcoholics' and brought within the treatment and intervention orbit individuals who would not otherwise have been considered as suitable cases for treatment. Thus new groups of women became potential clients of services. In addition, changing social attitudes towards women's drinking, rising alcohol consumption among women in the 1970s and increasing research on sex differences in vulnerability to alcohol provided a legitimate basis for demanding action regarding service responses to women with drinking problems (Camberwell Council on Alcoholism 1980; Thom 1994).

The demands for action on women's services came initially in the mid-1970s from a small group of activist researchers and practitioners allied to the Camberwell Council on Alcoholism in London. Largely women, they differed from nineteenth-century activists and philanthropists in the emphasis they placed on the need for gender-sensitive interventions. They pointed to the neglect of women in research studies, to the stereotyped images of women drinkers and to the inadequacy of existing services to respond to women's treatment needs. Active nationally and internationally for approximately seven years, the Camberwell group helped to establish Drugs Alcohol and Women Nationally (DAWN) as a network for information, research and action (Thom 1994). The group disbanded in 1980 with the publication of the first book to provide an examination of women's drinking in the UK (Camberwell Council on Alcoholism 1980). The issues raised in the book concerning the provision of appropriate services for women remain pertinent – and are still contentious today. They include questions about women's help-seeking behaviour for alcohol problems, the need for separate service provision for women and whether women do better with one kind of treatment approach rather than another.

Gender issues in help-seeking and service use

Reviews of women's help-seeking patterns have generally concluded that while women are more inclined than men to seek help for health or emotional difficulties, they are less likely than men to ask for help for alcohol problems (Beckman and Amaro 1984; Thom 1984; Smith 1992). The research literature concerning the 'barriers' to treatment entry for women is difficult to interpret. Few studies have examined the issues in any depth: they span a time period of approximately twenty years; they include samples of women drawn from different cultures and different social groups; most studies use samples of women who have entered treatment – thus missing those for whom the 'barriers' may have proved insurmountable; the studies lack standard or common measures and employ different theoretical approaches.

Attempts have been made to adapt theoretical models of health care utilisation to examine the use of alcohol services (see reviews by Jordan and Oei 1989; Smith 1992) and to develop a standardised instrument to identify barriers to treatment for addicted women (Allen 1994). But as yet these attempts have not resulted in a body of research theoretically and methodologically sound enough to draw firm conclusions from relevant to current circumstances. The poverty of research, both in terms of quantity and quality, is a major consideration in a review of the issues related to women's use of services. This is especially important if we try to extract conclusions which will be of practical value to the policy maker or service provider. Often the 'evidence' at our disposal is one or two studies conducted anywhere between 1970 and 1990, in the UK, Scandinavia, or more likely, the US. With those reservations in mind, there is widespread agreement regarding some of the factors which appear to influence women's help-seeking behaviour. Three areas which emerge from the available research are highlighted as especially important: failure to recognise the alcohol problem; the perceived costs of taking action; the perceived acceptability of available services.

Problem recognition

Failure to recognise harmful drinking may affect women more than men. The low representation of women in alcohol treatment services has been attributed to a combination of social factors which make it difficult for women to admit publicly that they are experiencing problems with drinking and difficult for service providers – such as general practitioners or social workers – to identify and respond appropriately to women clients.

Recognising and admitting to having a drink problem is difficult for men and women alike, but the stigma still attached to women's problem drinking may contribute to the greater reluctance of women to define themselves as problem drinkers – especially at an early stage when the risk of being labelled as 'alcoholic' may seem particularly threatening and inappropriate. In one recent UK study, over half of a sample of women felt that there was more social stigma attached to women's drinking than to men's (Mills-Hopper 1992). Another local study conducted in a London area reported that 90 per cent of the women and 83 per cent of the general practitioners surveyed agreed with the statement that excessive drinking in women is less tolerated by society (Williams and Gustafsson 1988). Even close family members may be unaware that a woman is experiencing problems. The difficulty of bringing the problem into the open is a major hurdle to help seeking. As one participant in a research study explained:

\ 'I certainly did not want to admit it ... it was also that I was telling so many lies and leading such a double life that it was too big to face ... I couldn't possibly tell my husband and actually when I did, he didn't believe me.'
(quoted in Thom and Edmondson 1989: 9) ∣ (

Some research indicates that women are more likely than men to report opposition to treatment entry from family and friends (Beckman and Amero 1984) or to experience less pressure to enter treatment (Smith 1992). On the other hand, compared to men, many women appear to have a shorter period of excessive drinking before seeking specialist help and it has been suggested that this 'telescoped' career is the result of greater family pressure to enter treatment (Camberwell Council on Alcoholism 1980).

Identifying the existence of a drink problem may be difficult for professionals as well as for the individual or family suffering from the problem.∣ Women tend to attribute their drinking problems to underlying causes – relationship problems, depression, or bereavement for instance – rather than interpreting alcohol use as a possible cause of their difficulties (Reed 1985; Thom 1986).∣∣ As a result, they may be more likely to seek help from agencies where the drink problem will be missed or misdiagnosed, or to present symptoms in a way which masks the association with alcohol. In one local survey, 64 per cent of women respondents agreed with the statement that it was more difficult for women to raise the subject of alcohol consumption with their doctor than it was for men (Williams et al. 1988).

Several studies have shown that professionals, even in the health and welfare services, often hold negative, stereotyped attitudes towards drinkers which make them reluctant to identify drinking problems (Shaw et al. 1978; Beckman and Amaro 1984; Thom and Tellez 1986) and less likely to consider alcohol as a factor in the symptoms presented by women (Smith 1992). However, work by Mowbray and Kessel (1986) suggested that doctors qualifying in more recent years may hold more positive attitudes towards the identification of alcohol problems among their patients; and the majority (88%) of general practitioners in the local survey quoted above said that they did not find it difficult to raise the subject with women patients (Williams *et al.* 1988).

We know even less about the attitudes and responses to problem drinkers of professionals other than general practitioners. Available studies seem to indicate that nurses and social workers at least suffer from similar difficulties to general practitioners and hold similar images of the woman drinker (Women's National Commission 1988; Wesson 1992) and that, in the workplace, referral for help with problem drinking is less likely among women employees than male employees (Smith 1992). The possible importance of coercion as a factor in treatment entry was considered by Allan (1987) in a study of attenders at an alcohol counselling service in Glasgow. She found that people referred from 'coercive' sources such as employers, the courts or hostels for the homeless, were more 'compliant' in regularity and continuance of attendance than referrals from non-coercive agencies. As women were under-represented in the coercive group, Allan speculated that this was one factor in their under-representation in specialist services.

Although all studies do not support the conclusion that women drinkers suffer greater social stigma than men (Beckman and Amaro 1984), the results from UK studies which illustrate the shame attached to women who are labelled as 'alcoholics', are replicated in studies from other countries (Gomberg 1988; Holmila 1991; Copeland and Hall 1992). They suggest that little may have changed in the fifteen years since the British Secretary of State for Social Services commented that, 'There is nothing manly or heroic or glamorous about those who drink too much. In men it is crude and embarrassing, in women it is plain sickening' (Ennals 1977).

The cost of help-seeking

Even once an alcohol problem is recognised, the perceived costs of taking help-seeking action may seem to outweigh the benefits. Work by Beckman and Amaro (1984) in the US lists the barriers women are likely to face when coming forward for treatment: financial costs; stigma; job-related and family-related costs; health and legal costs. There is, however, little research which examines women's own perceptions of the costs and benefits of entering treatment, or the actual costs experienced by those who do seek help.

Studies which have obtained the views of women entering treatment have generally reported fear of shame or loss of 'respectability' as a barrier to help-seeking. For example, among a sample of women entering treatment facilities in Australia, half reported delaying treatment entry because they believed there was greater social stigma attached to the woman drinker (Copeland and Hall 1992). Such fears appear to inhibit women's help-seeking approaches to generalist as well as specialist services. The study of Thom (1986) found that some women felt they might damage a good relationship with their general practitioner if they admitted to a drink problem. On the other hand, the results of the local study quoted above suggest that at least some general practitioners may be more approachable than their patients believe (Williams and Gustafsson 1988).

However, we do not as yet know whether current efforts to encourage the primary care team to expand their role in the provision of help for drinking problems will prove beneficial to women or result in earlier identification of women's drinking problems. Until recently, general practitioners and their patients have tended to see the general practitioner more as a gatekeeper to specialist services than as a provider of treatment and care within the general practice setting. Most patients believe that their problems are too trivial to take up the doctor's precious time (Thom and Tellez 1986; Williams and Gustafsson 1988; Thom et al. 1992).

Treatment entry may entail costs in the private as well as the public sphere. Some studies have indicated that relationships with a spouse or partner risk disruption when help for drinking problems is sought – because the dynamics of the relationship between partners, and in the family as a whole, may have adapted to accommodate the drinking behaviour. In the case of women, the partner is often a heavy drinker and may be unsupportive to the woman's help-seeking attempts. The findings from one UK study of women seeking help from an alcohol treatment unit illustrate the kind of difficulties women experience. Thirteen of the twenty-five women interviewed had lived or were living with a partner who was a heavy or problematic drinker; some had started drinking heavily to 'fit in' with their partners' leisure habits and friends; several reported attempts by partners to hinder help-seeking and encourage continued drinking. One woman quoted in the study told how, on her return from hospital, her husband had put a bottle right in front of her, poured it out and put it into her hands (Thom 1986). Similar findings have been reported in other studies (Camberwell Council on Alcoholism 1980; Beckman and Amaro 1984; Holmila 1991; Smith 1992).

Much of the discussion of costs has centred around women's fears that in entering treatment they may risk losing their children. The need to be a 'supermum', the fear of evoking a punitive rather than a helping response if social services or health professionals are approached, is reported in the research literature and anecdotally by many professionals. A survey conducted by the UK Women's National Commission in the late 1980s illustrated the strength of the problem. Just over half of a sample of Social Service Departments stated that they would encourage mothers with young children or pregnant women to come forward for help and many departments stressed that substance abuse *per se* would not be a reason for taking children into care. However, one department noted a marked reduction in the number of female clients referred over the previous months which seemed to coincide with extensive media coverage of the dismissal of an appeal by a drug-using mother whose baby was taken into care. A comment from another social service department concluded that the appeal decision had made a trusting relationship between the department and women more difficult (Women's National Commission 1988).

In the UK, despite recent moves by local authorities to develop policy statements concerning action towards the children of drug and alcohol misusing parents, women still fear the loss of children if they admit to an alcohol problem and they are especially reluctant to consider residential treatment if their children will be taken into temporary care. Attempts in some states in the US to introduce restrictive legislation on alcohol use by pregnant women and to bring pregnant women known to be heavy drinkers into custodial care have been criticised as a primitive approach, fundamentally unfair to women and likely to drive them away from prenatal care and treatment (NCADD 1990).

A major criticism of alcohol treatment services has been that they have developed without due consideration of the needs of women. One exploratory study of UK service providers' views on the problem of implementing gender-sensitive services indicated lack of child care; public stigmatisation of women; male-dominated agency settings; the attitudes of male (and to a lesser extent female) staff; female managers; and gender-insensitive publicity material as the main difficulties (Waterson and Ettorre 1989).

A recent survey of drug and alcohol services for women in the UK found that nearly a quarter of all agencies provided no specific services for pregnant women or women with children, that only half provided home visits, and that crèche/nursery facilities and women-only sessions had declined over the previous two years. The specific needs of different groups of women (elderly, Black, disabled etc.) were not recognised by most agencies (DAWN 1994).

In the earlier survey undertaken by the Women's National Commission, fewer than half of the district health authorities and social service departments reported any specific provision for women with substance use problems, and evidence given by the Ethnic Counselling Network to the Commission again highlighted the lack of appropriate services for Black and Asian women (Women's National Commission 1988). Other work has indicated that factors related to more general patterns of help-seeking may also be important in encouraging – or discouraging – use of specialist services. Marsh and Miller's review (1985), for instance, indicated that women from lower socioeconomic groups were likely to feel estranged from institutionalised sources of help and turn to more informal helping networks as a first resort; research undertaken largely in the US, suggests that specialist services may not be the most appropriate way to meet the needs of elderly people (Alcohol Alert 1988).

Despite considerable discussion of the importance of employing female staff and offering the choice of a female counsellor to women, there is no firm research evidence that this will attract or retain more women in treatment. Allan (1987, 1989) examined referrals to Glasgow Council on Alcohol to see whether a service providing many of the features suggested as particularly appropriate for women would succeed in attracting and retaining women clients and whether the service would reach a different type of clientele. The studies conducted by Allan found that although Councils on Alcohol appeared to be more successful in attracting female clients, the sex of the counsellor had no effect on treatment compliance for men or women, for the time clients remained in treatment or for the number of sessions they attended; furthermore, there were no significant differences in patterns of help-seeking between clients attending Glasgow Council on Alcohol and those attending an Alcohol and Drug Treatment Unit in the same city (Allan 1987, 1989). Allan (1989) concluded from her research that, despite the barriers posed for them, women appeared to be just as persistent as men in seeking out and receiving treatment.

Other research has reported a number of agency characteristics which may have an influential role in attracting women clients. Beckman and Amaro (1984), in their study of services in California, found that agencies with a higher proportion of female clients were more likely to report initial referral sources as advertisements and walk-ins. The same study reported that agencies offering after-care services and treatment for children were attended by significantly more women than agencies not providing those services. A study conducted in Australia comparing a specialist women's service with two traditional mixed sex services, found that the women's service attracted significantly more lesbian women, women with dependent children, women sexually abused in childhood and women with a maternal history of substance dependence (Copeland and Hall 1992). The UK survey by DAWN (1994) also identified a number of key factors which were associated with higher proportions of women attending services. These were the provision of a telephone help-line staffed by women; the provision of a specialist service for younger women; links with women's groups; local advertising of services; links with general practitioners and other health workers.

Summarising their review of the literature and the findings from their own study, Beckman and Amaro came to the conclusion that:

> The meagre data collected to date do not allow final conclusions regarding the specific nature of treatment barriers. However, patterns in our own data and in past studies clearly indicate that social support networks, societal norms, and the structure of treatment agencies promote inequities in the provision of services to women with alcohol-related problems.
>
> (1984: 341)

The precise nature of the inequities and the measures which might be taken to provide more woman-friendly services are likely to vary within different social and cultural contexts. It is not possible to extract from the existing research variables which can be generalised to all circumstances. A review of needs in relation to provision is a task which requires both national and local examination, and which would benefit from the inclusion of a consumer as well as a provider assessment of need.

Treatment modalities and outcome

While some consideration has been given in the research literature to the influence of service structures and staffing on attracting women into treatment, there has been very little attempt to examine gender differences in responses to different treatment modalities or treatment approaches (Henderson *et al.* 1982). The outcome of treatment has been the focus of more attention, although reviews of existing research have been hampered both because the differential effects of treatment on men and women are obscured through the reporting of aggregated data, and because many studies have too few women for separate analysis. Equally, interpretation of the research on women and treatment suffers from the same methodological problems as beset the field as a whole. To take just one example, drinking 'outcomes' may be measured in terms of abstinence, improved drinking, or quantity of alcohol consumed before and after treatment; outcome measures may or may not include a variety of 'life style' or quality of life dimensions including occupational, family or leisure dimensions (Thom *et al.* 1994). However, despite the difficulties in coming to any firm conclusions, existing studies have furthered our understanding of the importance of gender on treatment continuance and outcome and have provided some clues as to why women and men may respond differently to treatment.

Early studies of the effectiveness of treatment tended to conclude that women had a poorer prognosis than men. Writing in the 1950s Lincoln Williams, a prominent psychiatrist in the addiction field, described the:

> immature female psychopathic addict, often emotionally labile and a possible suicidal risk, perhaps sexually frigid, perverse or promiscuous ... the woman patient so vulnerable to emotional disturbances finds it more difficult to readjust her life and to make a successful recovery than the male.
>
> (Williams 1956: 9–11)

On the whole, early studies focused on the influence of patient characteristics on treatment outcome: the dependent woman, seen as more disturbed and more socially 'destroyed' than her male counterpart, was considered to have a poorer treatment prognosis. By the 1980s, this was being challenged as a stereotype unsupported by reviews of the research literature (Annis and Liban 1980; Vannicelli and Nash 1984) and attempts were underway to provide more appropriate services. Conclusions regarding similarity of treatment outcome for women and men in the short term – 3 to 12 months – were confirmed in a more recent review of twenty studies published between 1953 and 1992 (Jarvis 1992). However, the review also found that in the longer term – over 12 months – women were more prone to relapse (Jarvis 1992). Factors such as low support from a partner, the trauma associated with sexual abuse, low self-esteem, lack of physician involvement in after-care, lack of community involvement, and the greater occurrence of life-problems such as mental breakdown and ill-health have been suggested as possible explanations for gender differences in relapse (MacDonald 1987; Ellis and McClure 1992; Jarvis 1992).

Is there a need for specialist women's services and women-only approaches?

The literature on women's services provides ample anecdotal evidence that many women feel they benefit from separate women's groups or separate programmes within treatment agencies. The following quotations illustrate the views of some female clients who perceived a need for women's groups:

'I think there ought to be men only spaces for men and women only spaces for women ... because I don't think women talk so openly in a mixed group. I think they get into the supporting thing, supporting men with their problems. And male alcoholics judge women alcoholics – I have come across it – the double standards.'

(quoted in Thom and Edmundson 1989: 18)

'I became dependent on alcohol when I was about nineteen. I was living up north and working in a factory in a little town in Cumbria. I didn't like it at all – I found it depressing and I was also having problems coming out as a lesbian. I had been in a relationship for about two years and things were going on the rocks at this stage. I really needed to talk with other lesbians but I was isolated.'

(quoted in Wolfson and Murray 1986: 17)

'I was relieved to have a woman counsellor and feel that I couldn't have let myself trust a man in the same way'.

(quoted in Baker 1992: 52)

The research literature provides support for the contention that the needs of women entering alcohol treatment may differ from that of men (see Chapter 7). Studies of women's experiences of physical and sexual abuse (discussed in Jarvis 1992), of affective and phobic disorders (Allan 1991), and of stress disorders following traumatic events such as rape (Bollerud 1990), point to the importance of treatment approaches which take account of the social context of women's lives.

However, the extent to which women want or need separate provision remain contentious. In a study of psychological symptoms, psychiatric disorder and alcohol dependence amongst men and women, Allan (1991) challenges explanations of women's special treatment needs as lacking empirical support. In her study of attenders at a community-based voluntary agency and at an Alcohol Treatment Unit (ATU), she found no difference between men and women in the self-report of psychological symptoms by questionnaire. A small sub-group of women attending the ATU suffered from affective and phobic disorders and fulfilled 'the stereotype of the anxious, depressed female alcoholic', but Allan concluded that they were not typical of the majority of women in either sample.

Again, anecdotally, comments from women participating in a workshop discussion (Thom and Edmundson 1989) indicate that women, themselves, are likely to have mixed reactions to women-only groups or programmes, and to share the views of those who commented:

'In my case, I was brought up with four brothers ... I got on better with my father. I couldn't work there [in a woman-only rehabilitation unit]. I felt an oddity in a woman's only group.'

'I think it is also important that you learn how to relate to a man right from the start.'

(ibid.: 18–19)

As discussed in the previous section, changes in service structures and approaches appear to have some success in attracting
'hard to reach' groups into treatment, but their effectiveness in
terms of outcome is less clear. Research which has compared the
treatment outcome of women in specialist women's services with
women in mixed-sex institutions has produced contradictory
results. In some cases the benefits have been reported (Dahlgren
and Willander 1989); in others women are reported to do as
well in mixed-sex facilities (Duckert 1987; Copeland and Hall
1993). Copeland and Hall, in a comparative study of 80 women
in a special women's service and 80 women in two mixed-sex
services, found no significant difference in outcome between the
two groups. Since researchers have rarely been able to randomly
allocate women to different types of services, the element of
consumer choice – by attending or staying away from a particular
service – may colour findings on outcome. However, the conclusions drawn by Copeland and Hall (1993) remain pertinent: they
argue that it is important to move beyond the simple provision
of women-only services to consider the effectiveness of different
types of treatment, to look more closely at the content of treatment and to take account of the importance of interpersonal
interaction. If a particular treatment approach is less effective for
women, then the introduction of a women's section is merely icing
on the cake (ibid.).

The evidence for different treatment approaches

There is little empirical evidence supporting the benefits of one
type of treatment approach rather than another. The review by
Jarvis (1992) noted that the types of treatment associated with
better outcomes for men incorporated psychotherapy, milieu
therapy and attendance at Alcoholics Anonymous, a self-help
group. Better outcomes for women have been associated with
behaviour therapies and with programmes aimed at moderation
(Popham and Schmidt 1976; Sanchez-Craig et al. 1991).

Overall the literature suggests that women are less likely than
men to benefit from brief interventions (Bien et al. 1993). Brief
intervention trials in a general practice setting have been found
to be more effective for men than women (Scott and Anderson
1990; Anderson and Scott 1992). Another study of patients
referred to a hospital outpatient clinic, found that, relative to men,

women may benefit more from extended treatment (Robertson *et al.* 1986). Two large-scale studies in general health care settings found that women showed a reduction in drinking when given information and assessment feedback, with or without additional advice (Scott and Anderson 1990; Babor and Grant 1992). Sanchez-Craig *et al.* (1991), in a study which included 61 men and 35 women, found that the women benefited more when brief intervention was aided by a self-help manual. The authors speculate that women may welcome the greater responsibility for self-change. They also suggest that women may be more motivated to overcome their problem because of the fear of becoming stigmatised.

The experience of physical symptoms may also be a motivational factor. In the study by Sanchez-Craig *et al.* (1991), the women reported more symptoms for drinking compared to the men; women experiencing a greater number of symptoms required less therapist contact to achieve successful outcome – suggesting that adverse physical symptoms were a motivational factor which reduced the need for therapist activity. Work by Sokolow and colleagues (1980) found that positive outcomes in women were linked to programmes with a medical orientation, which may also indicate the influence of physical symptoms on motivation to complete treatment.

The influence of the therapist on treatment outcome, frequently discussed as probably influential on outcome, has been neglected in research studies. Encouragement given by women staff has been identified as an influence on outcome (Wiens and Menustik 1983); and the attitude of the therapist towards women drinkers has been suggested as the most critical aspect of treatment (Gomberg 1993). Sanchez-Craig and colleagues (1991) found that, although there was a tendency to achieve better outcome with same-sex therapist, the experience of the therapist was a more important predictor: more experienced therapists had a lower drop-out rate, perhaps because of their greater experience or perhaps because older therapists had greater credibility in the eyes of their clients.

Generally, involvement in group therapy, especially in mixed-sex groups, has been regarded as problematic for women. Women may feel less comfortable in mixed-group settings because they feel exposed to social judgements about the woman drinker, because they are less skilled or less at ease than men in coping with group dynamics, and because they are likely to be in the minority (Cronkite and Moos 1984). They are likely to feel inhibited in discussing topics around sexuality, sexual abuse and relationships with men and may find themselves cast in the traditional caring roles – supporting the recovery of men in the group while neglecting their own. A review by Baily (1990) quotes findings which indicate that women-only groups are associated with positive outcomes: women approach support groups differently to men, using them to deal with life-related issues rather than alcohol issues alone. The same review noted a superior outcome for women participating in group sessions compared to those assigned to individual, consultation-only sessions.

It is difficult to draw any firm conclusions from existing research on predictors of treatment outcome, or on the response of women to different treatment programmes. The point is often made that women are a heterogeneous group and that we need to examine more carefully the importance of factors such as age, ethnicity, socioeconomic background, disability, or support networks on treatment outcome and long-term rehabilitation. Although agencies are aware of the importance of adapting services to meet the needs of different groups of women (DAWN 1994), service development still relies on the observation, experience, and faith of agency staff rather than on monitoring or research procedures to point to the way forward.

SERVICES FOR WOMEN: THE WAY FORWARD?

In the ten years since DAWN published its first report on services for women in London (DAWN 1984), there have been considerable changes in awareness of women's treatment needs and of the importance of gender-based factors in help-seeking and treatment outcome. Although the most recent DAWN report (1994) still highlights areas where services in the UK appear to be failing to attract women or to offer appropriate responses, it also reflects a growing diversity in service provision aimed to meet the needs of women with drinking problems. Services offered now include a telephone help-line staffed by women, counselling for sex abuse, help for lesbian couples, women-only training courses, home visits, and a range of alternative approaches to child care – provision of a crèche, child care outside the specialist agency, domestic support and a baby-sitting service. Awareness of the possible links between gender variables, service structures and treatment content and delivery have informed these developments. At the same time, recent changes in the funding and delivery of community care, have threatened the existence of women-only rehabilitation services which cater for some of the most severely alcohol dependent women (Alcohol Concern 1994). The higher relapse of women over a longer time-frame highlights the importance of after-care and rehabilitation. Since the cost of providing specialist women-only services is likely to limit their availability, ensuring the development of gender-sensitive approaches in mixed-sex facilities and in generalist services is vital.

The swing towards early intervention and towards less intensive community approaches to care – characteristic of service development in the alcohol field as a whole – is also clearly visible in the recommendations for future development of women's services. As the target group for intervention has widened over the years to include people who are less excessive or damaged drinkers, so the role of primary care and generic health and social workers has become more important. Because of the association between alcohol and other problems, women (and men) are likely to present to a diverse range of helping agencies – social services, marriage guidance, the police and probation service, health care workers in the hospital and primary care sectors. The DAWN report (1994) stresses the need for funders and purchasers of services to look critically at all generalist services to ensure that they positively attract women. In a climate which emphasises health promotion and early intervention, it is necessary to convince generalist workers to incorporate gender-sensitive approaches to dealing with client's and patient's alcohol problems if women are to be reached in the earlier stages of harmful drinking. Targeted outreach work, which has grown in popularity over recent years, may also help to reach women who would not otherwise contact services.

Despite these apparently positive changes towards greater diversity in treatment approaches and service delivery, without appropriate research there is no way of knowing whether current trends and developments in service provision will secure better treatment outcomes for women. Monitoring of service use and research which includes the 'consumer' perspective is still lacking. Equally, there is a lack of research which examines the gender-based drinking and treatment experiences of men. The effort to redress the earlier imbalance in the literature towards men has resulted in many assumptions being made about the differences between women and men which demand closer examination if services are to become truly gender sensitive.

In an era when research and treatment services concentrated largely on the more severe 'alcoholic' drinker, it was perhaps possible to compare women as a group to men as a group. The acknowledgement that gender is an important factor in the response to problem drinking was an important step forward; but the future development of appropriately targeted services will require more careful 'matching' which takes account of the inter-action between gender and other variables.

REFERENCES

Advisory Committee on Alcoholism (1978) *The Pattern and Range of Services for Problem Drinkers*, Department of Health and Social Security and the Welsh Office, London: HMSO.

Alcohol Alert (1988) *Alcohol and Ageing*, A commentary by NIAAA Director, Enoch Gordis, Rockville, Md: National Institute on Alcohol Abuse and Alcoholism, US Department of Health and Human Services.

Alcohol Concern (1994) *Women's Residential Services Update*, London: Alcohol Concern Services Development Unit.

Allan, C. A. (1987) 'Seeking help for drinking problems from a commu-nity-based voluntary agency. Patterns of compliance amongst men and women', *British Journal of Addiction*, 82: 1143–47.

Allan, C. A. (1989) 'Characteristics and help-seeking patterns of atten-ders at a community-based voluntary agency and an alcohol and drug treatment unit', *British Journal of Addiction*, 84: 73–80.

Allan, C. A. (1991) 'Psychological symptoms, psychiatric disorders and alcohol dependence amongst men and women attending a commu-nity-based voluntary agency and an Alcohol Treatment Unit', *British Journal of Addiction*, 86: 419–27.

Allen, K. (1994) 'Development of an instrument to identify barriers to treatment for addicted women, from their perspective', *The International Journal of the Addictions*, 29 (4): 429–44.

Anderson, P. and Scott, E. (1992) 'The effect of general practitioners' advice to heavy drinking men', *British Journal of Addiction*, 87: 891–900.

Annis, H. M. and Liban, C. B. (1980) 'Alcoholism in women: treatment modalities and outcomes' in O. J. Kalant (ed.) *Alcohol and Drug Problems in Women*, vol. 5, Recent Advances in Alcohol and Drug Problems, New York: Plenum.

Babor, T. F. and Grant, M. (eds) (1992) *Project on Identification and Management of Alcohol-Related Problems. Report on Phase II: A Randomised Clinical Trial of Brief Interventions in Primary Health*

Care, Geneva: World Health Organization.

Baggott, R. (1990) *Health, Politics and Social Policy*, Aldershot: Avebury.

Baily, S. (1990) 'Women with alcohol problems: a psycho-social perspective', *Drug and Alcohol Review*, 9: 125–31.

Baker, S. (1992) 'Alcohol services and women' in *Women and Alcohol*, a national conference arranged jointly by the Department of Health and the Royal College of General Practitioners, 2 December 1991, London: HMSO.

Beckman, L. J. and Amaro, H. (1984) 'Patterns of women's use of alcohol treatment agencies' in S. C. Wilsnack and L. J. Beckman (eds) *Alcohol Problems in Women*, New York: Guilford.

Bien, T. H., Miller, W. R. and Tonigan, J. S. (1993) 'Brief interventions for alcohol problems: a review', *Addiction*, 88: 315–36.

Bollerud, K. (1990) 'A model for the treatment of trauma-related syndromes among chemically dependent inpatient women', *Journal of Substance Abuse Treatment*, 7: 83–7.

Breeze, E. (1985) *Women and drinking: an enquiry carried out on behalf of the Department of Health and Social Security*, London: HMSO.

Camberwell Council on Alcoholism (ed.) (1980) *Women and Alcohol*, London: Tavistock Publications.

Copeland, J. and Hall, W. (1992) 'A comparison of women seeking drug and alcohol treatment in a specialist women's and two traditional mixed-sex treatment services', *British Journal of Addiction*, 87: 65–74.

Copeland, J. and Hall, W. (1993) 'A comparison of a specialist women's alcohol and other drug treatment service with two traditional mixed-sex services: client characteristics and treatment outcome', *Drug and Alcohol Dependence*, 32(1): 81–92.

Cronkite, R. C. and Moos, R. H. (1984) 'Sex and marital status in relation to the treatment and outcome of alcohol patients', *Sex Roles*, 11: 93–112.

Dahlgren, L. and Willander, A. (1989) 'Are special treatment facilities for female alcoholics needed? A controlled 2 year follow-up study from a specialised female unit (EWA) versus a mixed male/female treatment facility', *Alcoholism Clinical and Experimental Research*, 13 (4): 499–504.

DAWN (1984) *Survey of Facilities for Women Using Drugs (Including Alcohol) in London*, London: DAWN.

DAWN (1994) *When a Crèche is not Enough. A Survey of Drug and Alcohol Services for Women*, London: Drugs and Alcohol Women's Network, GLAAS.

Duckert, F. (1987) 'Recruitment into treatment and effects of treatment for female problem drinkers', *Addictive Behaviour*, 12 (2): 137–50.

Ellis, D. and McClure, J. (1992) 'In-patient treatment of alcohol problems. Predicting and preventing relapse', *Alcohol and Alcoholism*, 27(4): 449–56.

Ennals, D. (1977) Speech given at the opening of the Health Education Council's North East Campaign on Alcohol Education. DHSS press release, 7 November.

Glatt, M. (1982) *Alcoholism*, Sevenoaks: Hodder & Stoughton.

Goddard, E. (1991) *Drinking in England and Wales in the Late 1980s*. An enquiry carried out by Social Survey Division of OPCS on behalf of the Department of Health in Association with the Home Office, London: HMSO.

Gomberg, E. L. (1988) 'Alcoholic women in treatment: the question of stigma and age,' *Alcohol and Alcoholism*, 23: 507–14.

Gomberg, E. L. (1993) 'Women and alcohol: use and abuse', *Journal of Nervous and Mental Disease*, 181 (4) 211–19.

Henderson, D. C. and Henderson, S. C. (1982) 'Treatment of alcoholic women' *Journal of Addictions and Health*, 3: 34–48.

Holmila, M. (1991) 'Social control experienced by heavily drinking women', *Contemporary Drug Problems*, Winter: 547–71.

Jarvis, T. J. (1992) 'Implications of gender for alcohol treatment research: a quantitative and qualitative review', *British Journal of Addiction*, 87: 1249–61.

Jellinek, E. M. (1976) 'Drinkers and alcoholics in ancient Rome', *Journal of Studies on Alcohol*, 37 (11): 1718–41.

Jordan, C. M. and Oei, T. P. S. (1989) 'Help-seeking behaviour in problem drinkers: a review', *British Journal of Addiction*, 84: 979–88.

Kelynack, T. N. (1902) 'Alcohol and the alcoholic environment in its relation to women and children', *The Medical Temperance Review*, V: 195–205.

Litman, G. (1975) 'Women and alcohol: facts and myths', *New Behaviour*, 24a (July): 126–9.

MacDonald, J. G. (1987) 'Predictors of treatment outcome for alcoholic women', *International Journal of the Addictions*, 22 (3): 235–48.

Marsh, J. C. and Miller, N. A. (1985) 'Female clients in substance abuse treatment', *International Journal of the Addictions*, 20: 995–1019.

Massot, P., Hamel, D. and Deliry, P. (1956) 'Alcoolisme feminin donnes statistiques et psychopathologiques', *Journal of Medicine*, 327: 265–9.

Mills-Hopper (1992) *Alcohol Concern: Women and Alcohol – A Research-based Evaluation*, London: Mills-Hopper Associates for Alcohol Concern.

Mowbray, A. and Kessel, N. (1986) 'Alcoholism and the general practitioner', *British Journal of Psychiatry*, 148: 697–700.

NCADD (1990) *Women, Alcohol, Other Drugs and Pregnancy*, New York: National Council on Alcoholism and Drug Dependence.

Plant, M. (1990a) *Alcohol Related Problems in High Risk Groups*, Geneva: WHO Publications.

Plant, M. (1990b) *Women and Alcohol: A Review of International Literature on the Use of Alcohol by Females*, Geneva: WHO Publications.

Popham, R. and Schmidt, W. (1976) 'Some factors affecting the likelihood of moderate drinking by treated alcoholics', *Journal of Studies on Alcohol*, 37: 868–82.

Reed, B. G. (1985) 'Drug misuse and dependency in women: the meaning and implications of being considered a special population or minority group', *International Journal of the Addictions*, 20 (1): 13–62.

Robertson, I., Heather, N., Dzialdowski, A., Crawford, J. and Winton, M. (1986) 'A comparison of minimal versus intensive controlled drinking treatment interventions for problem drinkers', *British Journal of Clinical Psychology*, 25: 185–94.

Roman, P. M. (1988) *Women and Alcohol Use: A Review of the Research Literature*, Rockville, Md.: US Department of Health and Human Services.

Sanchez-Craig, G. M., Spivak, K. and Davila, R. (1991) 'Superior outcome of females over males after brief treatment for the reduction of heavy drinking: replication and report of therapist effects', *British Journal of Addiction*, 86: 867–76.

Scott, E. and Anderson, P. (1990) 'Randomized controlled trial of general practitioner intervention in women with excessive alcohol consumption', *Drug and Alcohol Review*, 10: 313–21.

Shaw, S., Cartwright, A., Spratley, T. and Harwin, J. (1978) *Responding to Drinking Problems*, London: Croom Helm.

Smith, L. (1992) 'Help-seeking in alcohol-dependent females', *Alcohol and Alcoholism*, 27 (1): 3–9.

Sokolow, L., Welte, J., Hynes, G. and Lyons, J. (1980) 'Treatment-related differences between female and male alcoholics', *Journal of Addictions and Health*, 1: 42–56.

Thom, B. (1984) 'A process approach to women's use of alcohol services', *British Journal of Addiction*, 79: 377–82.

Thom, B. (1994) 'Women and alcohol – the emergence of a risk group', in M. McDonald (ed.) *Gender, Drink and Drugs*, Oxford: Berg.

Thom, B. and Berridge, V. (1995) *Special Units for Common Problems: the Birth of Alcohol Treatment Units in England*, Social History of Medicine, 8(1) 75–93.

Thom, B. and Edmondson, K. (1989) *Women, Family and Drugs: Women Talking. Report of a Workshop*, London: Commonwealth Secretariat.

Thom, B. (1986) 'Sex differences in help-seeking for alcohol problems – 1. The barriers to help-seeking', *British Journal of Addiction*, 81 (6): 777–88.

Thom, B. and Tellez, C. (1986) 'A difficult business: detecting and managing alcohol problems in general practice', *British Journal of Addiction*, 81: 405–18.

Thom, B., Brown, C., Drummond, C., Edwards, G. and Mullan, M. (1992) 'The use of services for alcohol problems: general practitioners and specialist alcohol clinic', *British Journal of Addiction*, 87: 613–24.

Thom, B., Franey, C., Foster, R., Keaney, F. and Salazar, C. (1994) *Alcohol Treatment since 1983: a Review of the Research Literature*, Report to the Alcohol Education and Research Council, London: The Centre for Research on Drugs and Health Behaviour.

Vannicelli, M. and Nash, L. (1984) 'Effect of sex bias on women's studies on alcoholism', *Alcoholism: Clinical and Experimental Research*, 8: 334–36.

Waterson, J. and Ettorre, B. (1989) 'Providing services for women with difficulties with alcohol or other drugs: the current UK situation as seen by women practitioners, researchers and policy makers in the field', *Drug and Alcohol Dependence*, 24: 119–25.

Wesson, J. (1992) *The Vintage Years: Older People and Alcohol*, Birmingham: Aquarius.

WHO (1992) *Woman and Substance Abuse 1992 Interim Report*, WHO/PSA/92.9, Geneva: World Health Organization.

Wiens, A. N. and Menustik, C. E. (1983) 'Treatment outcome and patient characteristics in an aversion therapy program for alcoholism', *American Psychologist*, October: 1089–96.

Wilson, P. (1980) *Drinking in England and Wales*, London: HMSO.

Williams, A. and Gustafsson, H. (1988) *Women and Alcohol: Lay and Medical Perspectives*, London: Tower Hamlets Association for Alcohol Services and Problems, Centre for the Study of Primary Care.

Williams, G. P. and Brake, G. T. (1980) *Drink in Great Britain 1900 to 1979*, London: Edsall.

Williams, L. (1956) *Alcoholism: a Manual for Students and Practitioners*, Edinburgh: Livingstone.

Wolfson, D. and Murray, J. (eds) (1986) *Women and Dependency*, London: DAWN.

Women's National Commission (1988) *Stress and Addiction Amongst Women*, London: Cabinet Office.

Chapter 9

Drinking problems among Black communities

Larry Harrison, Mary Harrison and
Victor Adebowale

INTRODUCTION

A search on the University of Hull's bibliographical database in
1994 yielded twenty-five pages of references on the prevalence of
alcohol-related problems among ethnic minorities. The literature
is voluminous, but it is almost entirely North American. There is
little in Europe and the UK to compare with this detailed study
of the prevalence, incidence and remission rates of alcohol dependence among ethnic minorities, nor of the differing patterns of
consumption and harm, service utilisation and treatment effectiveness.

Although some lessons can be learned from the American experience, the historical, cultural and demographic differences
between minority ethnic communities in the UK and North
America mean that American data have to be interpreted with
caution. It is necessary, therefore, to base any analysis of UK
problems on UK experience and research. In this chapter we
review the British literature on alcohol-related problems among
Black communities, before presenting recent evidence on mortality. We consider whether common assumptions about the extent
of problems in different ethnic groups are borne out by epidemiological evidence. Finally, we note the utilisation of treatment
services by Black people, before considering ways to improve
access.

This is, of course, a highly contentious subject. Although
Alcohol Concern, the UK national alcohol agency, has been
promoting debate about service access in recent years, many
service providers have been reluctant to acknowledge the need
to change established practices. Since they are personally free

from racist attitudes, they feel, there is no need to change organisational procedures. This is to misunderstand the nature of institutionalised racism.

> Institutionalised racism is not necessarily about people being nasty to one another. It is more about perpetuating traditional attitudes linked to the exercise of power – ignoring or rejecting other people's values and lifestyles, or ideas about illness and health, or about the social use of substances, because we assume that our ways are 'obviously' so much better, more civilised, more advanced, more scientific. It is about unthinking behaviour – or the refusal to think because it is easier and more comfortable not to.
>
> (Fernando 1993: 12)

Institutionalised racism is often about omission as much as commission; it is about the absence of attention to the particular experiences and needs of Black people within an organisation. In this chapter we consider some of the ways in which this ethnocentricity and neglect can be countered.

Throughout this chapter, 'Black' refers to those who are visibly different and who experience racism in Britain because of their visibility: those whose ethnic origins lie in the Caribbean, Africa, and the Indian sub-continent.

ESTIMATING PREVALENCE

The prevalence of alcohol-related problems among different ethnic groups can be estimated in a number of ways. It is possible to compare mortality amongst different country-of-birth groups for those disorders that are known to be alcohol-related, such as the alcohol dependence syndrome (ICD 303). In order to do this, crude death rates have to be standardised for age and gender, to take account of the different demographic characteristics of migrant groups.

It is also possible to calculate the extent of alcohol-related health, social and inter-personal problems directly from cross-sectional surveys, and indirectly from hospital admission statistics and by estimates of the proportion of minority populations drinking at higher risk levels.

There have been few specific studies of alcohol-related problems amongst Britain's Black population, and those that exist have concentrated on men born in the Indian subcontinent. There is relatively little evidence on the scale of alcohol-related problems among people of African descent, or amongst other ethnic groups such as Asian, Caribbean and Chinese people. In the following section we review indirect and direct estimates of alcohol-related harm, before considering the evidence from mortality data.

Indirect estimates

Indirect estimates of levels of alcohol-related problems have been made from cross-sectional surveys of alcohol consumption. The General Household Survey (GHS) has included questions on levels of alcohol consumption since 1978 and it is possible to analyse these data by country of birth. This analysis was conducted for all migrant groups by Balarajan and Yuen (1986) using 1978 data. When standardised for age and socioeconomic status in Britain, they found male drinking ratios of 103 for men born in England and 131 for men born in the North or South of Ireland. The drinking ratio for men from the West Indies was only 52 and that for men from the Indian subcontinent only 45, indicating much lower consumption levels than the UK national average.

There are several reasons for believing this to be a considerable under-estimate of alcohol consumption levels among minority ethnic groups, apart from the obvious fact that these data are over 15 years old and do not reflect current consumption patterns. First, as noted above, country of birth is not synonymous with ethnic origin, and although it is possible to sample second-generation migrants by examining parents' country of birth this analysis was not undertaken by Balarajan and Yuen. The data only refers to first-generation migrants, therefore, although over 40 per cent of Britain's current Black population were born in the UK (Bhat et al. 1988).

Second, the GHS is a household-based sample, and excludes those living in insecure accommodation. Yet any investigation of the health and social problems facing ethnic minorities in Britain must take account of tenure (Harrison et al. 1993). Ethnic minorities are more likely to be found in private rented accommodation in Britain and more likely to be lacking amenities like baths and inside WCs (OPCS 1993). It is precisely amongst these disadvantaged groups that the highest levels of problems are found in every community (Harrison et al. 1993).

Third, questions on weekly alcohol consumption may not be readily understood by those for whom English is a second language. This could include some members of Asian communities, particularly those who arrived in more recent years from Bangladesh, as well as the Greek and Turkish Cypriot communities, and some European, Middle Eastern, African and Chinese groups. There may also be considerable reluctance to disclose sensitive information to an unknown, probably White, official.

Moreover, the recommended risk levels described in Chapter 3 are of limited utility in comparative studies of this kind. Risk levels are likely to be different for population sub-groups. Alcohol-related harm occurs at lower consumption levels among the very young and the very old (Cahalan and Room 1974), among different ethnic groups and probably (although this has yet to be fully investigated) among different social classes. In a study of 147 alcohol-dependent inpatients, men born in the Indian sub-continent were found to have significantly higher values for gamma glutamyl transpeptidase (GGT) than White men with similar alcohol consumption levels. This suggests that Asian men may be more vulnerable to alcohol-related liver damage than the indigenous White population (Clarke *et al.* 1990), whether for predominantly environmental and sociocultural reasons (Harrison and Carr-Hill 1992) or for genetic reasons (Reed 1985).

Additional data on alcohol consumption among African-Caribbean men and women and on Gujarati Hindu, Sikh and Muslim men and women are available from surveys of blood-pressure, diabetes, diet and cardiovascular risk factors. These were reviewed by McKeigue and Karmi (1993). Although these surveys either do not report frequency distributions or do not use standard risk levels the overall picture appears to be the same: these ethnic groups report lower alcohol consumption levels than the native British.

While self-reported consumption data would have to be used in the absence of anything else, it is a very poor indicator of levels of alcohol-related harm. It assumes that there is a fixed relationship between levels of consumption and levels of harm that holds across communities, yet the epidemiological evidence shows this not to be the case. Mean alcohol consumption and rates of cirrhosis are poorly correlated between countries, for example, or even between regions in the same country, and it is also possible that there are variations in vulnerability by age, class and ethnicity

(Cahalan and Room 1974; Crawford *et al.* 1985). People also vary in their willingness to disclose drinking habits, with heavier drinkers under-reporting (Kreitman 1977). For this reason, most self-report surveys account for only a proportion of the alcohol known to be consumed from other sources. The 1978 OPCS study of drinking behaviour, for example, accounted for only 60 per cent of the alcohol known to be consumed from Customs and Excise statistics (Wilson 1980).

Direct estimates

Direct estimates of alcohol-related problems depend on cross-sectional surveys. The 1988 OPCS survey of drinking behaviour in England and Wales included questions about the adverse consequences of consumption, from which it appears that 6 per cent of men and 4 per cent of women could be considered problem drinkers, in that they had experienced two or more alcohol-related problems in the past three months (Goddard and Ikin 1988). The OPCS surveys do not examine ethnic status, however, and their surveys suffer from the same limitations as the GHS in that they both omit transient populations and, as noted above, may not be readily understood by those for whom English is a second language.

The main source of data on morbidity amongst ethnic groups is hospital admission statistics. These are based on a help-seeking population, known to be a minority of those with alcohol-related problems. Cochrane and Bal (1989) examined psychiatric hospital admissions by country of birth. Rates for alcohol-related diagnoses, calculated per 100,000 population, were extremely high for men and women born in Ireland and Scotland, whether first or all admissions were considered. Rates were also elevated for men and women from India. They were relatively low for those born in the Caribbean and very low for those from Pakistan.

Cochrane and Bal found an upward trend in alcohol-related admissions since 1971, with the highest increase (121 per cent) amongst men born in India. Admissions for Caribbean-born men had increased by about 75 per cent over this ten-year period, in line with the increase for men born in England. And although the Caribbean admission rate of 27 per 100,000 population in 1981 was less than that found for men born in England (38), it was considerably more than the 4 per 100,000 reported for the West

Indies (Burke 1984). Cross-national differences in hospital admission rates may reflect the availability of beds, or different admission policies, or the availability of provision in the community, both at a formal and an informal level, rather than differences in prevalence.

Some confirmation for Cochrane and Bal's findings comes from Mather and Marjot (1989), who found high rates of admissions for alcohol-related disorders within one psychiatric hospital for men born in India. Banerjee and Virdee (1986) noted higher than expected histological diagnoses of alcoholic liver disease among Asian men, based on the liver biopsies carried out by one London teaching hospital over a six-year period. There is known to be high prevalence of alcohol dependence in general medical settings, however, and because of sample bias most of the studies based on hospital or general medical populations cannot be used to estimate prevalence levels in the community.

Three specific community-based surveys have been conducted, by Burke (1984), Ghosh (1984) and Cochrane and Bal (1990). Ghosh (1984) interviewed 64 Asian men and 43 Asian women selected at random from general practitioner lists in Manchester and Liverpool. Ten per cent of the men were either drinking at high-risk levels (over 50 units per week for men and 35 units for women) or diagnosed as alcohol dependent. Ghosh did not employ a White comparison group, but these rates of heavy drinking would not be exceptional in the Northern region, where men drink more than the UK national average (OPCS 1990a).

The only specific survey data on drinking problems among African-Caribbean people is derived from a subset of Burke's (1984) epidemiological study of 243 West Indian migrants and 682 indigenous White British in Birmingham. This subset consisted of 43 West Indian and 93 British women. When these women were asked about the drinking behaviour of their husbands it appears that West Indian men were marginally more likely to drink heavily but asymptomatically. Four per cent of both West Indian and British men were reported to have family or work problems associated with alcohol. A further 7 per cent of West Indian men and 3 per cent of British men were said to drink 'excessively with intoxication'. None of the West Indian husbands were said to have psychiatric symptoms associated with excessive alcohol consumption whereas such symptoms were reported for 2 per cent of British husbands. Burke's survey relies upon partners' reports of drinking behaviour, however, and these may not be unbiased.

Cochrane and Bal (1990) conducted a community survey of 800 Sikh, Hindu, Muslim and White men selected at random from general practitioner lists in the West Midlands. Sikhs were most likely to be regular drinkers, followed by Whites and Hindus. Amongst both Sikhs and Hindus alcohol consumption was heaviest among older men, reversing the usual inverse relationship between age and consumption levels. Alcohol related problems were positively associated with consumption levels for all groups, but the very few Muslim men who drank alcohol consumed the most on average, and had the highest rates of problems.

These data cannot explain the over-representation of Indian-born men in psychiatric hospital admission statistics for alcohol-related disorders found in Cochrane and Bal's earlier (1989) study, even allowing for the fact that country of birth is not same as ethnic origin and that up to 10 per cent of those born in India could come from White British backgrounds (Cochrane and Bal 1990). The marked differences in hospital admission rates between African-Caribbean, Asian, Irish, Scottish and English men could reflect differences in help-seeking behaviour, or in the response of primary health care staff to different ethnic groups, rather than differences in prevalence.

Mortality

Marmot *et al.* (1984) calculated mortality ratios for causes likely to be alcohol related (cirrhosis, liver cancer, motor vehicle accidents and accidental drowning) for men and women born in Ireland, the Caribbean and the Asian sub-continent. While cirrhosis mortality rates were elevated for men from the Asian sub-continent (255) and from Ireland (204) they were lower than the national average for Caribbean-born men (91). Deaths from cirrhosis were below average for Asian and Caribbean-born women, but raised for Irish women (198). Data were restricted to the years 1970–72, however, and the numbers of deaths in some categories were extremely small: there were, for example, only thirty-six Caribbean men certified as dying from chronic liver disease and cirrhosis during this period. With such small numbers, death rates are unstable and may fluctuate considerably from year to year. Numbers were somewhat larger for deaths from motor vehicle accidents and accidental drowning, but less than 40 per cent of these deaths can be attributed to alcohol, making them less reliable as indicators of alcohol-related harm.

Balarajan *et al.* (1984) calculated mortality ratios for men and women of Indian descent, identified by the names on death certificates. Thirty-seven men and seven women died from chronic liver disease and cirrhosis in a sample of 3,657. Rates of death were much higher than expected for Punjabis (282) and Gujuratis (213) but were also raised for Moslems (161). Viral hepatitis, which can lead to chronic liver disease, is endemic in the Indian subcontinent but the concentration of cirrhosis mortality amongst males indicates that excessive alcohol consumption is the probable cause of raised mortality rates. Again, as liver disease is relatively infrequent the small numbers involved in this and similar studies mean that rates are unstable and may fluctuate considerably over time.

Recent trends in mortality

A consistent finding from UK studies of migrant health in the 1980s was that rates of alcohol consumption and related harm appeared to be substantially lower for African and Caribbean men than for the native British, but raised for men born in the Punjab. This is not what would be expected from a comparison with US data, where Black Americans have substantially higher alcohol-related mortality than Whites (Herd 1989).

One of the main sources of UK data on alcohol-related mortality by place of birth dates from 1979–83, however (OPCS 1990b); the frequently quoted standardised mortality ratios for different ethnic groups (Marmot *et al.* 1984) are based on data from 1970–72. These data are now over twenty years old, and there is evidence that alcohol-related problems are increasing more rapidly in some ethnic groups than in the general population (Cochrane and Bal 1989). McKeigue and Karmi (1993), in a recent review of the literature, concluded that it would be useful to monitor secular trends in alcohol consumption for ethnic groups. This is particularly necessary among Africans and Caribbeans, they argue, since an increase in alcohol consumption in a group that already has elevated morbidity rates for hypertension and stroke would pose a serious risk to health.

In order to up-date estimates of alcohol-related harm among ethnic groups, Harrison *et al.* (1994) examined mortality among those born in the Caribbean (Barbados, Jamaica, Trinidad and Tobago, Guyana and other Caribbean islands); Ireland (Irish Republic); and the Indian sub-continent (Bangladesh, India and Pakistan). As in Chapter 3, cirrhosis was taken as an indicator variable, and all diagnoses for chronic liver disease and cirrhosis (ICD-571) were considered, rather than diagnoses with a specific mention of alcohol (ICD-571.0–571.3), because of evidence of substantial under-reporting of specified alcoholic cirrhosis (Haberman and Weinbaum 1990). It is probable that up to 80 per cent of all cirrhosis mortality is the consequence of heavy alcohol consumption (Schmidt 1977).

Unpublished data were obtained from the OPCS for mortality from specific causes by country of birth. The number of deaths from chronic liver disease and cirrhosis (ICD 571) over the three years 1989–91 were aggregated in order to increase sample size, and standardised for age and gender for each country of birth group, using population data from the 1991 census (OPCS 1993). The results are shown in Table 9.1.

The data reported in Table 9.1 indicate that cirrhosis rates for all three minority groups are elevated. In contrast to studies undertaken in the 1970s, those born in the Caribbean no longer appear to be in an advantageous position: there are now more deaths from cirrhosis than would be expected. These findings are subject to the same caveats that apply to the earlier study by Marmot and colleagues: the numbers of observed deaths

Table 9.1   Mortality in England and Wales from chronic liver disease and cirrhosis (ICD 571) in different place of birth groups, 1989–1991

Place of birth	Standardised mortality ratio	Number of deaths
All	100	9,188
Irish Republic	222*	359
Indian sub-continent	164**	236
Caribbean	113***	77

Source: (Harrison et al. 1994)

Note: 95 per cent confidence intervals: *195.8–252.2, **140.8–192.5, ***85.9–148.4

Mortality for the Irish and Asian groups is clearly elevated, as the lower limits of the confidence intervals are well above 100. The picture for the Caribbean is less clear, as the confidence intervals are rather wide.

are relatively small (though larger than in prior studies) and statistically unstable. The authors plan to combine data on cirrhosis with those for all alcohol-related mortality, therefore, in order to increase sample size and improve the reliability of the prevalence estimates. They also plan to analyse trends in these data over time.

Given the scale of this problem for Black communities, access to effective treatment services is a national priority. The indications are, however, that Black people are under-represented among the users of mainstream services. In the following section ways to improve access to alcohol treatment services are considered.

SERVICE ACCESS

There are two principal strategies available to service providers: the creation of specialist Black agencies, and the enhancement of existing services. In the following section we consider each of these strategies in turn.

Some of the arguments for separate service provision for Black people with alcohol problems will be familiar, since they have also been advanced in relation to other services. Housing, health and social services have consistently failed to provide services which are accessible to, and cater for the particular needs of Black people (Rooney 1981; Dominelli 1988; Roys 1988). There appears to be a similar situation in the alcohol field. It is not uncommon for alcohol agencies to see very few Black clients: 40 per cent of agencies surveyed for the London Alcohol Forum in 1990 had no African-Caribbean service users at all (Russell *et al.* 1991).

One agency helping people with substance problems, the Bridge Project in Bradford, undertook a specific study into the low rate of service uptake in an area with many potential Asian clients (Patel 1993). Only 1 per cent of the service users were Black compared to 20 per cent of the local population. Many potential service users did not know of the existence of the agency. Those who knew of the agency said they did not use it as they assumed it to be a White-run agency, catering for White clients. This assumption was based on their dealings with other health and welfare services in the area: 'Asian people told us that agencies did very little to make their services inviting to them, both in terms of physical appearance and service provision' (Patel 1993: 42). Most expressed a preference to talk to an Asian counsellor as they felt that they would be understood better, and although there were some who wished only to speak to a White counsellor, as they were afraid that confidentiality would be difficult to maintain in a close-knit Asian community, it appears that on the whole Black people find it easier to approach a Black organisation when they are experiencing difficulties.

There are several reasons why this might be the case. First, Black clients feel that they are unlikely to encounter racism from within a Black organisation. Allied to this, there may also be an assumption among Black service users that it is safe to let down their guard: for many, wariness is a necessary survival strategy when dealing with White authority figures. Feeling safe may also make it easier for a Black client to establish trust, engage with the agency and form a therapeutic relationship with agency staff.

Many Black people seeking help from a White facility will feel in a difficult position, and some feel additionally vulnerable in that help-seeking may confirm their own feelings of powerlessness and appear to corroborate negative stereotypes of Black people as being problematic and unable to solve their own problems. In short, Black service users are placed in the position of being the passive recipients of White peoples' help. The fact that in a Black agency the responsibility for organising Black people is undertaken by Black people avoids this problem and, more than this, offers validation to Black people in that they can be seen to be dealing with their own problems themselves.

Separate organisations are also in a position to speak with a distinct voice, articulating the particular position of Black service users and making clear demands on their behalf. Furthermore it could be argued that as Black people are over-represented in the 'misery' statistics of homelessness, prison and mental health problems (Bhat et al. 1988) they need to be represented in the 'solution' statistics. A separate Black organisation can provide more information about Black drinkers and may be able to offer opportunities for research to be conducted from a Black perspective, by researchers who are part of the Black community and who are identified with their needs and interests (Harrison, M. 1993).

Black agencies could also help to influence the training of social workers and other professionals, for example by providing training to develop understanding of the impact that racism can have on the everyday lives of Black people and the way in which it affects their life opportunities. As a result Black agencies can become part of the broader context in which Black people challenge, and support themselves in challenging, racism.

Black individuals in mainstream organisations often face isolation either as service users or as staff members and they may expend an inordinate amount of effort in dealing with and trying to overcome this isolation. One of the routes taken by organisations who need to establish a profile as offering services to Black people is to recruit one Black worker who is expected to find a large Black constituency – often without support, or in the absence of a developed and clear organisational policy. This approach is essentially tokenistic. The Black member of staff is usually of junior rank and is subject to scrutiny by senior management. At the same time, partly because of the Black workers' low position in the hierarchy, other staff members are resistant to learning from them and the organisation often finds it difficult to make any changes advocated by them.

Current thinking mitigates against the employment of one Black person in this way, since they are essentially placed in a double bind situation, in which they are both supposed to bring about substantial change in the organisation while at the same time not 'rocking the boat' or causing disruption. (An example of this kind of contradiction is provided by Profitt 1986 in his discussion of Race Adviser posts.) Black managers in White organisations also face particular problems due to status contradiction: that is they have low status through being Black and high status because of their managerial position.

Black agencies need to be 'Black' in the political sense: that is catering for people who are visibly different and who experience racism in Britain because of their visibility. There is also a need for agencies to employ Asian workers who speak the languages of the communities they are serving and with whom Asian service users can identify (Patel 1993). Hopefully, Black centres for people with alcohol problems could provide some choice for groups of different ethnic and cultural backgrounds. At the same time there needs to be awareness of the impossibility of catering for all possible ethnic and cultural differences. It is not feasible for any single worker to have a detailed knowledge of all the different cultures they might encounter in a busy inner-city agency, although it is possible for them to have an open attitude to cultural difference.

Despite these reasons for providing separate services for Black people, many argue that it is not a viable option. First, because there may be particular difficulties in obtaining funding. Black agency organisers may have more limited access to organisational networks and may lack friends in high places. Black agencies tend to be small and recent changes in legislation, particularly the National Health Service and Community Care Act 1990, is having a profound effect on the voluntary sector (see Chapter 10). Smaller agencies are at a disadvantage in this situation, in that they may find it more difficult to get specialist workers to do the policy work that is essential for development and resource acquisition. Without adequate funding Black agencies may be 'set up to fail'.

Second, Black people are tax-payers and therefore have a right to access mainstream services. There is the possibility that mainstream service providers could use the existence of an alternative as an excuse not to develop their own service for Black people (Dominelli 1988).

Third, some advance the argument that separate Black services are a form of apartheid, playing into the hands of racists who argue that multi-racial services cannot work.

It is not necessary to pose the case for widening access to mainstream services as an alternative to the development of separate Black provision, however. Rather we can recognise that both approaches are valid and necessary, with differing local situations determining which is most appropriate. Two brief accounts, the first of a mainstream agency which succeeded in widening access to Black service users and the second of a recently established separate Black agency, indicate the particular and often overlapping concerns of these two approaches in practice.

Patel (1993) offers a valuable account of how a mainstream agency dealing with substance-abuse problems (predominantly illicit drugs) undertook development work in order to increase access for Black clients. A survey of the local population revealed that it was predominantly Asian, but comprised of several different cultural groups – between them speaking nine different languages, belonging to three main religious groups, and coming from three different generations.

After consultation with the community it was decided to work initially with the largest and most accessible group, young Pakistani men. Outreach work was conducted in mosques and with Asian elders as well as with youths. Information and counselling sessions were held in health centres, GP surgeries and Black community centres. An ongoing programme of training was instituted to equip all agency staff to work with Black clients. Culturally sensitive advertising and information was developed by the agency, and gradually, over 18 months, confidence began to build amongst the local Black population, who made use of the agency's services increasingly. Hyare (1994) has also shown the importance of forging an alliance with key individuals in the local community, and building on their ideas and experience, to design culturally sensitive alcohol education.

Patel draws some general conclusions for mainstream agencies wishing to widen access for Black and other ethnic minority clients:

- Ongoing outreach work is essential to discover the needs of the community, build trust and maintain awareness of changing needs.
- There is a need to employ Black workers to gain credibility and trust, and to attract Black people to the service. However, it is also important that these Black workers work with all clients, Black and White, and possess appropriate specialist skills; they should not be employed in a tokenistic fashion.
- It is vital to employ Black staff at all levels of the organisation as well as seeking adequate representation on management committees. It is equally important that Black people are involved at a policy-making level in order to ensure that policies are racially and culturally sensitive and that Black people do have the opportunity to effect change at management level.
- As far as possible the make-up of the staff team should reflect the cultural diversity of the local population.
- It is important that all staff in the agency receive training to work with Black clients and it is vital that the training is an ongoing process, not a one-off 'race awareness' session.
- Advertising needs to be culturally sensitive and not just translated from existing material in English. Use should be made of Black newspapers and Black radio programmes.

In 1993, *Choices*, an agency offering a service for Black people with alcohol problems, was set up in Stockwell, South London, under the auspices of the Alcohol Recovery Project. Three full-time staff, a manager, two social workers and a half-time administrator were appointed and the agency became operational in April 1994. During the first six months, April–September, there were 111 continuing client contacts and an equal volume of one-off, predominantly telephone enquiries.

A significant number of clients reported that either they had had bad experiences of seeking help elsewhere or that they had been unable to find help. The numbers of clients in the second six-month period of operations increased, and it was necessary, unfortunately, to turn some potential clients away since the current staffing levels could not meet the demand. At the time of writing (1994), there has not been time to conduct a detailed analysis of the work, but initial impressions indicate that service users have a number of undiagnosed mental health problems, as well as cases of diagnosed mental health problems where the alcohol component of the problem has not previously been recognised. A proportion of service users also have problems with illicit drug use, predominately with cannabis and crack cannabis.

Innovative outreach work is being conducted by the agency in conjunction with the Afro-Caribbean Mental Health Association and with housing agencies. Counselling services are being provided on a regular basis at local GP's surgeries. It should be noted, however, that much of this outreach work is being provided on a voluntary basis by the agency staff as there is insufficient funding. Current funding from the local health authority is for a three-year term and the agency has been given 'priority group' status. Future plans to continue to develop the work and to engage more staff to meet the existing demand inevitably depend on local health authority funding decisions: for Black services these decisions have an additional political dimension as well as a service one.

To summarise: recent analysis of alcohol-related mortality by country of birth indicates that problems are greater than expected among Black communities in Britain, and appear to be on the increase. This is particularly serious because there are also indications that Black people are less likely to use alcohol treatment services. Two strategies to improve access to services have been considered in this chapter: enhanced access to mainstream services, and the creation of separate agencies run by and for Black people. Both approaches are needed. Given the fact that the Black population in Britain is widely dispersed there could never be enough specialist services to meet the total need, even if this were desirable. Black people must have access to mainstream agencies. Separate Black agencies have a vital role in creating the impetus for change, however. In addition to providing a service for hard to reach groups, specialist Black agencies have an important role as research and demonstration projects, in which culturally sensitive and anti-racist approaches can be developed.

REFERENCES

Balarajan, R., Adelstein, A. M., Bulusu, L. and Shukla, V. (1984) 'Patterns of mortality among migrants to England and Wales from the Indian sub-continent', *British Medical Journal*, 289: 1185–7.
Balarajan, R. and Yuen, R. (1986) 'British smoking and drinking habits: variations by country of birth', *Community Medicine*, 8(3): 237–9.
Banerjee, A. and Virdee, S. (1986) 'Alcohol-related problems in ethnic minorities', *British Journal of Psychiatry*, 149: 383.
Bhat, A., Carr-Hill, R. and Ohri, S. (eds) (1988) *Britain's Black Population*, (2nd edn), Aldershot: Gower.
Burke, A. (1984) 'Cultural aspects of drinking behaviour among migrant West Indians and related groups', in N. Krasner, J. S. Madden and R. J. Walker (eds) *Alcohol Related Problems*, New York: Wiley.
Cahalan, D. and Room, R. (1974) *Problem Drinking Among American Men*, New Brunswick, NJ: Rutgers University.
Clarke, M., Ahmed, N., Romaniuk, H., Marjot, D. H. and Murray, L. I. M. (1990) 'Ethnic differences in the consequences of alcohol abuse', *Alcohol and Alcoholism*, 25(1): 9–11.
Cochrane, R. and Bal, S. (1989) 'Mental hospital admission rates of immigrants to England: a comparison of 1971 and 1981', *Social Psychiatry and Psychiatric Epidemiology*, 24: 2–11.
Cochrane, R. and Bal, S. (1990) 'The drinking habits of Sikh, Hindu, Muslim and white men in the West Midlands: a community survey', *British Journal of Addiction*, 85(6): 759–69.
Crawford, A., Plant, M. A., Kreitman, N. and Latcham, R. W. (1985) 'Self-reported alcohol consumption and adverse consequences of drinking in three areas of Britain; general population studies', *British Journal of Addiction*, 80: 421–8.
Dominelli, L. (1988) *Anti-Racist Social Work*, London: Macmillan.
Fernando, S. (1993) 'Race, culture and substance problems', in L. Harrison (ed.) *Race, Culture and Substance Problems*, Hull: University of Hull.
Ghosh, S. K. (1984) 'Prevalence study of drinking alcohol and alcohol dependence in the Asian Population in the UK', in N. Krasner, J. S. Madden and R. J. Walker (eds) *Alcohol Related Problems*, New York, NY: Wiley.
Goddard, E. and Ikin, C. (1988) *Drinking in England and Wales in 1987*, London: HMSO.
Haberman, P. W. and Weinbaum, D. F. (1990) 'Liver cirrhosis with and without mention of alcohol as cause of death', *British Journal of Addiction*, 85(2): 217–22.

Harrison, L. and Carr-Hill, R. (1992) *Alcohol and Disadvantage amongst the Irish in England, London*: Federation of Irish Societies.

Harrison, L., Carr-Hill, R. and Sutton, M. (1993) 'Consumption and harm: drinking patterns of the Irish, the English and the Irish in England', *Alcohol and Alcoholism*, 28(6): 715–23.

Harrison, L., Sutton, M. and Gardiner, E. (1994) *Secular Trends in Cirrhosis Mortality among First Generation Migrants to England*, Hull: University of Hull.

Harrison, M. (1993) 'Substance problems: an anti-racist perspective', in L. Harrison (ed.) *Race, Culture and Substance Problems*, Hull: University of Hull.

Herd, D. (1989) 'The epidemiology of drinking patterns and alcohol-related problems among US Blacks', in *The Epidemiology of Alcohol Use and Abuse among US Minorities*, Research Monograph No. 18 Washington, DC: National Institute on Alcohol Abuse and Alcoholism.

Hyare, I. S. (1994) 'Ethnic dimensions', *Alcohol Concern Magazine*, 9(4): 14–5.

Kreitman, N. (1977) 'Three themes in the epidemiology of alcoholism', in G. Edwards and M. Grant (eds) *Alcoholism: New Knowledge and New Responses*, London: Croom Helm.

Marmot, M., Adelstein, A. and Bulusu, L. (1984) *Immigrant Mortality In England and Wales, 1970–78*, London: HMSO.

Mather, H. M. and Marjot, D. H. (1989) 'Alcohol-related admissions to a psychiatric hospital: a comparison of Asians and Europeans', *British Journal of Addiction*, 84(3): 327–9.

McKeigue, P. and Karmi, G. (1993) 'Alcohol consumption and alcohol-related problems in Afro Caribbeans and South Asians in the United Kingdom', *Alcohol and Alcoholism*, 28(1): 1–10.

Office of Population Censuses and Surveys (OPCS) (1990a) *General Household Survey 1988*, London: HMSO.

Office of Population Censuses and Surveys (OPCS) (1990b) *Mortality and Geography: a Review in the Mid-1980s*, The Registrar General's Decennial Supplement for England and Wales, series DS No. 9, London: HMSO.

Office of Population Censuses and Surveys (OPCS) (1993) *The Census, 1991: Country of Birth, Great Britain*, London: HMSO.

Patel, K. (1993) 'Ethnic minority access to services', in L. Harrison (ed.) *Race, Culture and Substance Problems*, Hull: University of Hull.

Profitt, R. (1986) 'The role of the race advisor', in V. Coombe and A. Little (eds) *Race and Social Work*, London: Tavistock.

Reed, T. E. (1985) 'Ethnic Differences in Alcohol Use, Abuse, and Sensitivity: A Review with Genetic Interpretation', *Social Biology*, 32(3/4): 195–209.

Rooney, B. (1981) 'Active mistakes: a grass roots report', in J. Cheetham, W. James, M. Loney, B. Mayor and W. Prescott (eds) *Social and Community Work in a Multi-racial Society*, London: Harper & Row.

Roys, P. (1988) 'Social services', in A. Bhat, R. Carr-Hill and S. Ohri (eds) *Britain's Black Population*, (2nd edn), Aldershot: Gower.

Russell, J., Baker, P., Hinton, T. and Philo, J. (1991) *Survey of Alcohol Needs and Services in London*, London: London Research Centre.

Schmidt, W. (1977) 'The epidemiology of cirrhosis of the liver: a statistical analysis of mortality data with special reference to Canada', in M. M. Fisher and J. G. Rankin (eds) *Alcohol and the Liver*, New York: Plenum Press.

Wilson, P. (1980) *Drinking in England and Wales*, London: HMSO.

Chapter 10

Community care policy and the future of alcohol services

Larry Harrison, Philip Guy and Wayne Sivyer

INTRODUCTION

New arrangements for funding community care were implemented in England on 1 April 1993. The objectives were set out in the White Paper *Caring for People* (Department of Health 1989). Government funding for social care was to be restructured with the intention of securing 'better value for taxpayers' money', and making agencies more accountable through the clarification of responsibilities. The government claimed the reorganisation would promote the development of domiciliary, day and respite services to enable people to live in their own homes whenever feasible, and would encourage the development of the independent sector (Department of Health 1989:5).

Treatment and rehabilitation for people with alcohol and drug problems was not central to the new legislation, the National Health Service and Community Care Act 1990, or the preceding White Paper, *Caring For People*; indeed in the latter document, alcohol and drug problems barely rate a mention. Because of the precarious nature of the funding arrangements for many of the non-statutory agencies providing alcohol or drug services, however, the community care reorganisation is likely to have far-reaching consequences – an issue that was debated at some length during the passage of the Bill through the House of Commons, and during the initial phase of the policy's implementation (see, e.g. House of Commons 1992).

This chapter examines the impact of government policies on health and community care on alcohol treatment services. First, the post-war development of alcohol policy is detailed, before describing the different ways in which two local authorities attempted to negotiate the changes in community care funding, and the unforeseen consequences for service delivery. Finally, changes in the policy process are outlined and the consequences for service development explored.

POST-WAR DEVELOPMENT OF ALCOHOL SERVICES

In the immediate post-war period, UK alcohol consumption was relatively low in volume, and alcohol-related harm was regarded by the government as a low priority; indeed in 1951 the Ministry of Health was reluctant to support the attendance of a British representative at a scientific meeting on alcoholism sponsored by the World Health Organisation (WHO) on the grounds that the problem was so minimal in England and Wales it hardly merited the appointment of one full-time consultant psychiatrist in the National Health Service (Robinson and Ettorre 1980).

The alcoholism sub-committee of the WHO's Expert Committee on Mental Health was established in 1950 and met on several occasions. It was critical of the almost universal lack of interest in alcohol dependence among member states and argued for the adoption of a range of treatment programmes, with in-patient care reserved for the most severe cases (WHO 1951). In an era when health policy was largely determined by expert opinion and professional consensus, the WHO sub-committee was extremely influential in raising the profile of alcohol-related problems. Its emphasis on treatment over prevention, and on a medical rather than a social response, supported those in the UK calling for the introduction of specialised services within the NHS.

The first NHS inpatient Alcoholism Treatment Units were established in the mid-1950s, and formed the core of service provision for two decades (Davies 1979). By the late 1970s there were thirty-two Alcoholism Treatment Units in England and Wales (Robinson and Ettorre 1980).

That the first facilities should have been hospital-based might seem surprising in retrospect. It is true that in the period when the units were established, professionally led institutionalisation was still the dominant form of service provision across client groups. However Alcoholism Treatment Units were, in the main, operated as a sub-speciality in large psychiatric hospitals and these hospitals were themselves due to close under community care plans published by the government in the same year as the first official policy statement on the treatment of alcohol dependence (Ministry of Health 1962a, 1962b). In addition, the WHO sub-committee had called for 'ambulatory' or outpatient treatment for the majority of patients (Robinson and Ettorre 1980).

In the early years of the NHS, however, policy development was largely incremental and clinician-led, and the drive to establish and expand specialist treatment was often due to the entrepreneurial activities of senior hospital doctors. At this time, the British government's policy was determined, for all practical purposes, by clinical practice and past precedent, rather than by any rational analysis of policy objectives and options.

Amongst the committed professionals who campaigned for the introduction of specialised hospital units, Glatt (1974, 1982) was arguably the most influential. Glatt established the first Alcoholism Treatment Unit at Warlingham Park Hospital, near Croydon, in 1951. Although not a member of the Ministry of Health Advisory Committee, he appears to have had a direct influence on government policy through the publicity which his work attracted (Robinson and Ettorre 1980).

Robinson and Ettorre (1980) trace the development of Alcoholism Treatment Units through three government policy statements. The first, *Hospital Treatment of Alcoholism* (Ministry of Health 1962b), advised Regional Hospital Boards to develop specialised inpatient units, modelled on Glatt's wards at Warlingham Park and St Bernard's Hospital, Southall: although outpatient clinics could be provided, treatment was to be a hospital-based activity.

Six years later, the memorandum *Treatment of Alcoholism* (Ministry of Health 1968), mentioned the term 'community' for the first time. A greater stress on the value of outpatient services was apparent, but community provision was not seen as an alternative to hospital treatment. For many in the alcohol field at this time, community-based services were assumed to be synonymous with 'after care' (Glatt 1974: 226). Good quality community-based services could reduce the length of hospitalisation that patients required, but inpatient care would continue to be essential (Glatt 1974: 225).

In the 1970s the incremental approach to policy and service development that characterised the early years of the NHS was replaced by corporate rationalism and a faith in rational planning techniques. The newly created Department of Health and Social Security (DHSS), itself the result of a Whitehall reorganisation designed to promote greater rationality and efficiency in government, began to take a more systematic approach to service planning, and the title of the third circular, *Community Services for Alcoholics*, (DHSS 1973), indicates the beginning of a policy shift. It followed the recommendations of a Home Office working party, that responsibility for 'habitual drunken offenders' should pass to the health departments and be integrated into a comprehensive treatment and rehabilitation service (Home Office, 1971).

Community Services for Alcoholics gave details of the financial assistance that was to be made available to non-statutory services to provide residential care and rehabilitation for problem drinking offenders. Six more Alcoholism Treatment Units were to be established and it was planned to increase the number until there was at least one 'within reasonable distance of every major centre of population' (DHSS 1973: para 3). For this to be an effective strategy, the DHSS acknowledged that there needed to be a complementary development of a range of community-based services.

Despite this commitment to a sizeable expansion of hospital inpatient care, the government was becoming concerned, at a time of increasing financial constraints, that the scale of alcohol-related problems was far greater than had been appreciated. Epidemiological research indicated that at least 400,000 people might be alcohol dependent in England and Wales (DHSS 1975). The model of treatment which had been advocated – inpatient psychiatric care based upon long-term group therapy – could not possibly form the basis for a national response to a problem of this magnitude. Most people with drinking problems did not receive specialist help, there were long waiting lists for inpatient treatment and dissatisfaction over the selection criteria operated by many Alcoholism Treatment Units. Few accepted homeless or offending problem drinkers, who were considered to have a poor prognosis. Because of growing criticism of service provision, the DHSS funded a pilot project to demonstrate how limited resources might be deployed more efficiently (Spratley *et al.* 1975, 1977; Shaw *et al.* 1977).

The success of the Maudsley Alcohol Pilot Project led to recommendations that primary health care, social work and probation staff should be given the support of a district-based specialist multi-disciplinary team, called the Community Alcohol Team, or CAT. The CAT's most important task would be 'not to provide specialised second level care to alcohol abusers but to educate and support those general agents giving primary care' (Spratley *et al.* 1977: 342). It was, the report concluded, a 'more valuable use of a specialist's time to spend an hour talking with the GP about an alcoholic patient than to see that patient himself in an outpatient clinic' (ibid.: 342).

The Maudsley Alcohol Pilot Project represents something of a watershed, in that almost all of the ideas which inform current UK practice either originate or feature prominently here: that is, the pre-eminent role of primary level 'community agents' – not just health care teams, but social workers, probation officers, religious leaders and voluntary workers; the analysis of why these agents may not feel confident in their dealings with problem drinkers; the need for better professional qualifying training; and the need for specialists to fulfil a supportive function (Spratley, 1975: 2941; Shaw *et al.* 1978: 764).

These ideas were endorsed in the White Paper *Better Services for the Mentally Ill* (DHSS, 1975) which argued that future emphasis should turn towards a locally-based treatment service. Specialist units were often located in remote mental hospitals, and, as local services developed, the 'role and location of these units would have to be reconsidered' (DHSS, 1975: 66). The scale of alcohol-related problems was such that it could not be met by a substantial increase in the number of hospital or community services – although the latter needed a 'great deal more development in some areas'. Instead, there needed to be a greater awareness on the part of all staff in the health and social services.

The White Paper reviewed the development of community services and concluded that it had been uneven and ill-coordinated, with local authorities often regarding provision for problem drinkers as lying outside the mainstream of residential care. A small number of hostels and rehabilitation units had been established in the 1950s and 1960s, largely by non-statutory agencies. These were often the only services working with homeless offenders, and the government hoped that the availability of DHSS grants, announced in the circular *Community Services for Alcoholics*, would encourage a major expansion. Funds were provided to voluntary agencies on a 'pump-priming' basis, with local authorities having to agree to assume an increasing share of the costs. This was intended to ensure that rehabilitation services would be 'absorbed into the pattern of statutory and voluntary residential care' (DHSS, 1975: 64).

Unfortunately, many local authorities were reluctant to accept long-term financial commitments, while others did not want hostels in their area because they feared it would attract difficult clients. The government was aware that if its plans were to be successful it would need to secure greater involvement from primary level staff in the health and social services, who appeared reluctant to work with problem drinkers (Shaw *et al.* 1978). Local authorities would need encouragement to support residential care, and a decision was awaited on the future role of regional Alcoholism Treatment Units. In order to examine these policy questions in detail, the DHSS appointed a multi-disciplinary Advisory Committee on Alcoholism (DHSS, 1975: 66). In a series of cogent and well-argued reports produced over the next four years, the Advisory Committee recommended a greater emphasis on prevention, better training for primary level staff, and a greater range of services for problem drinkers (DHSS and Welsh Office 1977, 1978, 1979). Alcoholism Treatment Units should become a resource for local communities, and no more hospital units 'of a regional character should be set up' (DHSS and Welsh Office 1978: s. 4.25).

Although the government never commented on these key proposals, it is clear that Alcoholism Treatment Units were no longer regarded as the core of alcohol services. The assumption underlying previous policy was that specialist hospital services needed to be developed, and primary level staff trained to recognise and refer patients: now primary level staff were expected to provide services, with support from community-based specialists.

This reversal of policy on treatment came as a result of a number of inter-related developments, including the growing emphasis on community as opposed to institutional care, pressure to enhance the role of the non-statutory sector, and demands for a greater public investment in prevention. And although some are sceptical about the impact that scientists can have on public policy, it is clear that throughout the 1970s the policy debate was influenced by research, especially on epidemiology and treatment evaluation (Edwards 1993). It became generally accepted that the scale of the problem was too great to be managed by specialist inpatient units, and that intensive hospital treatment was not demonstrably more effec-tive than brief intervention (Orford and Edwards 1977; see Chapter 6).

COMMUNITY SERVICES IN THE 1990S

While many Alcoholism Treatment Units continue to exist in the 1990s, the phasing out of large psychiatric hospitals has led to some units being closed and others becoming community-based agencies. Growth in community-based provision has been considerable, particularly in CATs, local advisory and counselling services, and residential care. By the mid-1980s there were fourteen multi-disciplinary CATs in England and Wales, based to a greater or lesser extent on the recommendations of the Maudsley Alcohol Pilot Project, and providing the main form of local statutory service (Alcohol Concern 1987; Clement 1987). There were sixty-nine Councils on Alcoholism, alcohol advisory services or similar non-statutory counselling agencies, and 1,350 branches of Alcoholics Anonymous (Alcohol Concern 1987). In April 1992, before the introduction of the community care reforms, 159 agencies were identified which provided residential care for people with substance problems who were on income support (MacGregor et al. 1993b). These included units specialising in crisis intervention, detoxification, nursing care and residential rehabilitation, as well as therapeutic communities. There were also over fifteen private clinics, which do not receive public funds and are not directly affected by the community care legislation (Alcohol Concern 1987).

With the exception of Alcoholics Anonymous, each branch of which is financially self-supporting, most non-statutory agencies are funded through small centrally administered budgets and specific grants which are usually administered locally by health authorities, either from money specially allocated or from general funds. One consequence is that projects are often short term, and large sums of money are wasted each time a service is reestablished when there is no continuity in funding. There is also a very real difficulty in recruiting high-calibre staff on short-term contracts and uncompetitive salaries.

The funding of residential agencies has always been particularly vulnerable. Before the implementation of the NHS and

Community Care Act, clients were referred to residential agencies by social workers, probation officers, family doctors, counsellors and others. Clients who qualified for income support were entitled to have a proportion of their fees paid by the Department of Social Security. The amount paid rarely covered the full cost and agencies had to seek 'top-up' fees from local authorities and other sources. Although this was not always forthcoming, the availability of government funding via the Department of Social Security gave the residential care sector a measure of stability which encouraged its growth.

Between 1979 and 1990 the cost of providing social security payments for residential care escalated from £10 million to £1,270 million, only a small proportion of which was due to an increase in the number of services for problem drinkers (Ogden 1992: 4). Pressure from the Treasury to reduce public expenditure made an attempt to gain control of this budget inevitable. Unlike the previous funding arrangements, which were open-ended, the 1990 Act placed the overall budget under Treasury control. Following the implementation of the Act, responsibility for paying for residential care rests with the local authority rather than the Department of Social Security. Essentially, the community care reforms represent a move from provider to purchaser-dominated services, and from institutional to community-based care. Local authorities become the lead agency in the purchase of care over a wide spectrum of need.

The initial impact of the legislation was monitored by MacGregor and colleagues (1993a, 1993b). In the first fifteen months of operation, the number of people with substance problems occupying registered beds declined by 23 per cent, from 2,009 to 1,546 (MacGregor et al. 1993b: 1). One-third of all clients did not complete the assessment procedure, 23 per cent waited over 10 days for assessment and over half waited more than ten days between referral and admission.

The residential sector suffered as a consequence. By the autumn of 1993, two agencies had closed, two more were due to close, and a number of others were 'struggling' (MacGregor et al. 1993b: 32). There was a 19 per cent reduction in the number of registered beds. Most agencies were having to adopt short-term economies, such as reducing staffing levels and leaving staff vacancies unfilled, and some were reducing the duration of their treatment programmes in response to market pressures. There was evidence that bargaining between purchasers and providers was intensifying, although many felt that local authority purchasers were handicapped by their lack of knowledge and skills in relation to the needs of people with drink and drug problems.

Many of the needs of the client groups covered by the new arrangements were already familiar to local authorities: for example, older people, people who have a disability, and people who have a mental disorder. People with alcohol problems had never been other than a peripheral concern for local authority social service departments, however. The requirement to assess the treatment and rehabilitation needs of people with alcohol problems was likely, therefore, to present local authorities with a major challenge. In order to illustrate the differing ways in which local authorities attempted to manage these changes, and the consequences for the overall quality of services for people with alcohol problems, we present the following case study.

IMPLEMENTATION IN TWO LOCALITIES

The new arrangements for community care are permissive rather than prescriptive. The ways in which local authorities may respond to service demands are many and various. Whilst this may give cause for concern in terms of equity, it does mean that approaches can be refined to meet local circumstances. Thus, while there are broad similarities in the general service arrangements for community care between individual authorities, there appears to be no standard preferred response to the everyday business of identifying and meeting the service needs of people experiencing alcohol or drug problems.

The precise nature of the new responsibilities for this client group under the NHS and Community Care Act 1990, and the extent of the changes necessary for local authorities to implement these reforms, were specified in the guidance document *Alcohol and Drugs Services and Community Care* (Department of Health 1993). This document was made available only three weeks before the Act became operative. This circumstance, coupled with an acknowledged lack of previous service experience in the field of substance problems, left many local authorities ill-prepared for their new task. This was clearly reflected in the absence of detailed or developed service proposals in respect of alcohol and drugs in many of the community care plans produced by local authorities for the period 1993–4.

In practice, a number of local authorities chose to delegate responsibility for identifying and meeting the service needs of people with substance-use difficulties to specialist, non-statutory agencies. MacGregor *et al.* (1993a: 42) found that 46 per cent of their sample of 108 local authorities had chosen this route. Others placed the task with the small number of specialist alcohol and drug workers within their own social services departments. A further group attempted to incorporate this task into the mainstream assessment and care management structures.

Two adjacent local authorities in the north of England provide an illustration of different approaches to the implementation of this particular aspect of the community care reforms. There is considerable variation between local authorities in their response to the National Health Service and Community Care Act, and these two authorities should not be taken as typical. They do, however, provide a detailed case study of the difficulties with which local government was faced, and the effect this had on the provision of non-residential services for people with alcohol and drug problems.

Case A is a county council which serves a population of some 850,000 across a wide geographic area, including inner-city, urban and rural settings. Data collected by the Regional Substance Misuse Database show that the prevalence of both alcohol and drug-related difficulties in this area is one of the highest in the region. Many practitioners believe the scale of these problems is explained by the presence of several seaports and a once dynamic fishing industry with a long-established tradition of heavy drinking, which has become part of local culture. The largest town in this county can be called Seaport. Within Seaport there are three agencies working specifically with substance-use issues, one public sector and two non-statutory, together with a NHS Alcoholism Treatment Unit that is on the verge of closure. Case A can be called Greater Seaport.

Situated in the other principal towns of Greater Seaport there are a further two statutory agencies, one of which offers inpatient detoxification, and three non-statutory agencies, one of which is a centre for residential rehabilitation. Although in principal two of the non-statutory agencies specialise in offering services to illicit drug users, in practice people with alcohol problems access these services as well. One of the main reasons for this is a lack of services in rural areas. This issue has been made a priority for service development, leading to a rapid expansion in rural outreach teams.

Case B is a Metropolitan Borough Council covering a smaller geographic area with a much smaller population than that of Greater Seaport. There are some 230,000 people living within the boundaries of this authority in a combination of urban and semi-rural communities. Historically, this is a region dominated by coal mining and allied industries, all of which have been in sharp decline over recent years. Case B can be called Coaltown. The reported incidence of alcohol-related problems and illicit drug use, whilst lower than that recorded in Seaport, is nevertheless substantial and growing. As in Greater Seaport, a high rate of alcohol consumption among people living in the area is attributed to the development of a local drinking culture which has an association with the presence of particular industries. There is just one agency providing services specifically for people experiencing substance-use difficulties. This agency, a joint venture between the local authority, the health authority and a non-statutory alcohol service, is able to provide a comparable range of services and facilitates to those on offer in the larger neighbouring county of Greater Seaport.

GREATER SEAPORT

In 1991 Greater Seaport initiated a programme of incremental change within its social service department, designed to conform with central government's timetable for the implementation of the NHS and Community Care Act (1990) while continuing to meet the requirements of the Children Act (1989). Generic neighbourhood social work teams, established some ten years previously, were replaced by provision directed towards identified client groups. In effect there was a complete separation of adult services from those for children and families, in terms of both management and practice.

The roles of assessment and resource provision were also separated. This was in direct response to the new community care arrangements which required the setting up of internal markets both within the NHS and local authority social service departments. Under the new community care arrangements, adult services are accessed through Community Care Teams (the purchasers) who are responsible for assessment, service procurement and overall care management. Where possible and practicable, the department's own service provision has been organised into a number of multi-purpose resource centres (providers) under separate line management. A major theme in Greater Seaport's development of community care procedures for adult services is the concept of 'single door' access, whereby designated assessment officers in the Community Care Teams undertake all needs assessments, including those involving substance-use problems, and Care Coordinators from these same teams manage and monitor all care plans. A direct consequence has been a reduction in the number of service access points across the county.

While Greater Seaport was, and remains, committed to this idea of 'single door' access, it was recognised early on that within the Community Care Teams there was likely to be a significant absence of direct experience in working with people presenting with alcohol problems. Interim measures were adopted, so that assessment and care management for this client group could be undertaken by the specialist social workers seconded to the local statutory alcohol and drugs agency, or by senior social work practitioners attached to mental health resource centres. This arrangement lasted for approximately ten months. During this period specific training was provided for the Community Care Teams by the specialist social workers. One year after reorganisation all but a handful of assessments were undertaken by these teams, with the specialist social workers acting in a supporting or consultancy role.

As part of the general management strategy, day-to-day responsibility for community care budgets was devolved to the managers of Community Care Teams. Whilst the alcohol and drug component of these devolved budgets was not ring-fenced it was accounted for publicly at a county level in a move designed to demonstrate a commitment to this particular client group. This practice was adopted in response to the expressed concerns of advocates and pressure groups, not least of which was a lobby of service providers. As no estimates of the numbers likely to seek access to services for alcohol and drug problems existed prior to the implementation of the reforms, Greater Seaport was unable to forecast budgets with any confidence. For the first year the expenditure limit for alcohol and drug services was set at around £385,000. In the event this sum proved more than adequate to meet demand, possibly because many clients who were already taking up beds retained their rights to social security payments for the first few months. Demands on local authorities are likely to be higher in 1994–95.

During the initial six months of community care some fifty assessments of individuals with substance-use difficulties were completed within Greater Seaport. In each instance, assessment followed a specific request for funding of a residential rehabilitation placement. (In the first two years of operation there were no examples in Greater Seaport of assessments being requested for any other reason.) Less than a quarter involved alcohol problems. While referrals originated from a variety of sources, one local non-statutory drugs agency was responsible for the majority. In part this can be attributed to the drug agency's involvement in a joint initiative with the local probation service aimed at identifying alternatives to custody. Many of the assessments involved illicit drug users facing court appearances.

In contrast, few of those presenting with alcohol problems were involved in current criminal proceedings. Referrals for this group came from medical practitioners and family members; there were also a large number of self-referrals, however – a far higher number than among the illicit drug users. In all but a small number of cases, where local community-based services were identified as more appropriate, the outcome of these assessments was a decision to fund residential rehabilitation as requested. Despite this agreement only a third of those assessed chose to take up offered placements and of these just four remained in such placements beyond twelve weeks.

The existence of a range of established community services within Greater Seaport for those experiencing problems with alcohol may partly account for the lower referral and take-up rate within this group. Access to these services remains largely unchanged by the new community care arrangements. These local services presently include the Alcoholism Treatment Unit. Admission to this NHS unit does not require the involvement of social services. With the closure of this unit expected within the next five years the possibility exists that residential provision for people with alcohol problems will become a more significant issue for Greater Seaport.

COALTOWN

As in Greater Seaport, Coaltown developed a phased response towards its new responsibilities in accordance with central government's timetable, whilst also developing services in line with the requirements of the Children Act (1989). In a similar move to that of its neighbour, Coaltown separated adult services from those for children and families, and sub-divided the functions of the former into purchasing and provision. Aside from alcohol and drugs services, which were not included in this reorganisation, access to all other adult provision follows a similar pattern to that of Greater Seaport. Responsibility for the management of the community care budget for substance problems was passed to one of Coaltown's Principal Officers for Children and Families, who, because of an arrangement which predates the community care reforms, was the line manager for the single social work practitioner attached to the local alcohol and drugs agency.

As before, there were no baseline figures to guide managers in setting a budget for this client group. After a brief, largely unhelpful, telephone trawl of residential rehabilitation units across the country to ascertain how many individuals from the area had been clients in these units in the previous twelve months, the budget was fixed and 'ring-fenced' at £75,000 for the first year. Once again, this figure proved to be an over-estimate of the actual demand.

In recognition of the possibility that one social worker would not be able to cover all of the work generated by the community care assessments, it was agreed that a nurse specialist, employed by the health authority, the only other statutory worker with the local alcohol and drugs agency, would undertake needs assessments and ongoing care coordination on behalf of Coaltown. In placing this responsibility with specialist workers, Coaltown also agreed to the development and implementation of separate assessment methods and procedures to those employed with other client groups. In practice this led to an initial filtering of requests for community care services, before moving on to the full assessment. As in Greater Seaport, requests all centred on residential rehabilitation.

In the first six months of community care, twelve assessments were undertaken within Coaltown. Again, less than a quarter related to alcohol. While referrals came from a number of sources the majority were referred by the probation service. In a similar pattern to that observed in Greater Seaport, this larger group consisted entirely of illicit drug users involved in current criminal proceedings. Funding of residential rehabilitation was agreed in every instance, though only five chose to take up arranged placements. Of those who did attend a rehabilitation unit, three left within the first week and the remaining two managed less than seven weeks.

Overall, these two examples, while demonstrating different approaches to the organisational practice of assessing the community care needs of people with alcohol or drugs difficulties, show remarkably similar outcomes. In both cases attempts to place individuals in residential rehabilitation have been generally unsuccessful. In both authorities, more money was spent conducting assessments than was spent on rehabilitation services. In addition, both authorities were confronted by a number of practical difficulties in implementing the new arrangements for this client group which had not been acknowledged or addressed adequately in either the formulation of the National Health Service and Community Care Act (1990) or the subsequent guidance, *Alcohol and Drug Services and Community Care* (Department of Health 1993).

Prior to the implementation of the new legislation, neither authority had any general experience in meeting the service needs of people with substance-use difficulties. Such work was seen as peripheral and the responsibility of a very small number of specialist practitioners. With the shift of priority brought about by the new community care arrangements, managers and generic social work practitioners were obliged to face this acknowledged lack of experience when confronted by the extraordinary range of competing beliefs, philosophies and treatment approaches which characterise the alcohol and drugs field.

Many of these approaches have never been the subject of formal independent evaluation, particularly in the field of residential rehabilitation, and the methods and practices of some units appear to run counter to accepted social work values. One qualified social worker, commenting on the approach taken by a rehabilitation centre, called it 'treatment through humiliation'.

This issue was further complicated by clients often expressing strong views about both the nature of their problem and the most appropriate service to meet their needs. Thus matching needs to services – whilst taking proper account of client choice – became a major problem for both authorities, made worse by an absence of accurate information about the range of service options and by the wide geographic spread of such provision.

Additionally, whilst some residential rehabilitation units have since changed their requirements, most insisted that clients be alcohol or drug free on admission. There is unfortunately little evidence from the two authorities to suggest that the NHS afforded any formal priority to requests for detoxification services in these circumstances. As a consequence, admission to a rehabilitation unit could be delayed, or alternatively a medical practitioner could determine, on clinical or resource grounds, that detoxification was inappropriate. In the early stages of the new arrangements, Greater Seaport was obliged to access detoxification services from the private sector in such circumstances. Similarly, where the outcome of an assessment indicated that local community services would be the most useful in addressing a client's identified needs, there was no evidence to suggest that community agencies gave any priority to referrals which were the result of a community care assessment. Finally, as previously noted, many of those seeking residential rehabilitation were facing court appearances. Frequently residential rehabilitation was seen as an alternative to custodial sentences by some service users and, perhaps, by the courts.

There was tension between agencies in both localities following the implementation of the community care legislation and the consequent changes in funding for residential rehabilitation. Both authorities believed assessment officers were being subjected to pressures to comply with the needs of the criminal justice system rather than the specific community care needs of the individual. In Greater Seaport the non-statutory agency involved in the Home Office diversion from custody project expressed, for its part, impatience at the length of time taken by the assessment procedure. The probation service, which had lost funding as a result of the community care reforms, believed that it was entitled to call on the local authority for a prompt and efficient assessment service. This difference of views, together with the emergence of competition for scarce resources, introduced a note of discord into the previously harmonious relations between probation, the non-statutory sector and the local authority social services.

The reasons given for the low take-up rate and the premature ending of placements were identical in both cases. Discussions with referrers, service providers and clients suggest that many placements do not occur, or end prematurely, because clients no longer felt they were necessary, found the placement unhelpful, received a custodial sentence, or simply disappeared. It should be emphasised that this does not necessarily mean that the clients difficulties had been resolved.

There are three possible reasons why the assessment procedure is not resulting in successful placements. The first is that the assessment process is not addressing the client's readiness to change or not giving weight to the source of expressed motivation – such as family difficulties or the threat of imprisonment. The second is that the process of needs assessment is overly bureaucratic and not client-centred. Placements fail, or are not taken up, because clients feel that they have no ownership of the process. The third possibility is that residential rehabilitation is not an effective intervention, even for those who request it, indicating that local community-based alternatives need to be developed as a matter of urgency.

In this context, specialist practitioners from both authorities expressed frustration, feeling they had been reduced to being gate-keepers to an expensive residential service. The amount of time devoted to community care assessments in the first few months in Greater Seaport meant that all other aspects of their specialist practitioners' work had to be abandoned. The direct provision of treatment and preventive services to a large number of problem drinkers and their families was replaced by what was felt to be a bureaucratic exercise on behalf of a small minority of clients requesting a high-cost service. In a sense, the 'tail was wagging the dog'.

Underlying this concern was a jaundiced view of residential rehabilitation as 'little more than a licence to print money'. One well-informed care manager from Greater Seaport viewed changes introduced by the residential sector – in terms of lower weekly charges and shortened therapeutic time scales – with a degree of cynicism. He believed that as the residential services were not local they were difficult to monitor, and that he, and many of his colleagues, had grave reservations about some of the oppressive practices within these agencies that they were being asked to sanction.

This is in stark contrast to the lengthy debate that parliament held on the performance of the residential sector, when the tone was overwhelmingly uncritical (House of Commons 1992). Faced with the choice of spending large sums of money on sending one client to a residential establishment of unproven effectiveness, or investing the same amount of money in community-based alcohol services which would reach a large number of clients, local care managers have begun to ask awkward questions. In the future the pressure for accountability, evaluation, and demonstrable cost-effectiveness may be difficult to resist.

THE FUTURE OF THE 'REHAB'

There was much debate in parliament during the passage of the National Health Service and Community Care Bill about the threat posed to the viability of residential services in the independent sector. The government met with trenchant criticism from back-bench MPs, and, in order to safeguard the passage of the Bill through the House of Commons, had to promise to 'ring fence' funding for alcohol and drug services – a commitment it later withdrew (House of Commons 1993).

It is understandable why many believed that alcohol and drug services should be exempt from the Bill's provisions, or given a protected status. Philosophically, residential services are somewhat out of kilter with the rest of mainstream community care provision: the former are about treatment and rehabilitation rather than care. The distinction may seem a narrow one, particularly if the objective of treatment is controlled drinking rather than the more common goal of total abstinence, but nevertheless the distinction is real. The majority of people calling on local authorities under the new arrangements are seeking a maintenance service rather than an agent of change.

In some ways however, the alcohol field has suffered as a result of its isolation, and there are advantages to be gained from closer integration into mainstream provision. Alcohol-related problems are often seen as peripheral to the work of social service departments and allocated to a very small number of specialist practitioners (see pp. 254–6 above, and Alaszewski and Harrison 1992). The need to develop expertise in assessment is forcing many social workers into a reassessment of priorities, and this may help to end the marginalisation of this client group within social services.

Other benefits may become apparent in the near future. The treatment philosophies of some residential rehabilitation units are idiosyncratic, if not therapeutically suspect, and many of the arguments centring on normalisation and deinstitutionalisation, used in the context of mainstream community care, would seem to apply. As Heather and Robertson point out:

> the absurd way to treat problem drinkers is to take them off to a residential institution miles away – physically or psychologically – from the home community. A drinking problem does not reside in the individual but arises from the interaction between the individual and his environment. If drinkers are to resist cues for drinking they must be in contact with the environment that conveys these cues.
>
> (1989: 283)

The purchaser–provider split is already creating pressures for the evaluation of cost-effectiveness. Some of the most expensive treatment programmes, in this country as in the US, are those for which there is least evidence of effectiveness (Holder *et al.* 1991), and a reappraisal of therapeutic practice in the residential sector is long overdue. The residential sector could also benefit from external scrutiny of its values and working philosophies. As MacGregor *et al.* point out:

> The assumption of responsibility by local authorities for these clients has introduced into service provision a new group of players who bring in different perceptions of need and good practice, who are willing to question established perceptions and knowledges, and who may draw on different values and work within a different culture.
>
> (1993a: xviii)

The need to retain the confidence of the purchasing authorities could act as a counterweight to the insular tendency of agencies and professionals in the alcohol field. It could also encourage more dialogue with social service departments, raising awareness of the needs of problem drinkers and promoting the development of new and innovative forms of service delivery. There is a recognition by some local authorities that alternatives to residential rehabilitation need to be found, and some are considering diverting part of their budget to fund more community projects (MacGregor *et al.* 1993b: 38). The non-statutory sector has nothing to fear from such developments. It has the flexibility to respond to new needs as they develop, and it is often more successful than statutory services in improving access for marginalised groups, like the homeless (see Chapter 5).

There is a danger, though, that pressures for cost-effectiveness, or cost containment, could restrict the non-statutory sector's capacity for innovation. Agencies might be obliged to offer low-cost interventions, and avoid the risks associated with originality. This could be reinforced if purchasers favour spot purchasing – seeking to reduce costs by placing clients in the least expensive programmes. Block purchasing deals, on the other hand, might disadvantage some of the smaller agencies by creating local service monopolies. There are already signs that the independent, not-for-profit sector is losing some of its autonomy, through contract compliance clauses, while larger, more entrepreneurial agencies are expanding at the expense of others. Competitive pressures could eventually lead to the survival of a handful of large, national agencies, with a consequent loss of client choice.

There are also problems arising from the geographical distribution of residential services. The present distribution has evolved in a haphazard way, rather than through any empirically based analysis of need. As a result, the availability of care often varies inversely with need, and there are large areas with no residential facilities. It has been suggested that a residential service may have to deal with clients from between forty to fifty different local authorities each year: 87.5 per cent of clients residing at Turning Point in North Tyneside, for instance, came from outside of the North Tyneside local government area (House of Commons 1992). More recent figures provided by MacGregor et al. (1993a) for the period immediately after the new arrangements for community care came into effect show a slight improvement:

> Of those cases referred to the residential sector in the three months April – June 1993, 74 per cent were previously residing outside the local authority area in which the agency itself was located while only 17 per cent had a last known address that was in the same local authority area as that of the agency itself.
>
> (1993a: xi)

The quasi-market created by the community care legislation is unlikely to achieve a geographical redistribution of services without government intervention. In future, the location of independent-sector residential services will be determined by market demand, that is, by the willingness or ability of purchasing authorities to pay. At present, the transitional funding grant is not distributed equitably, in that some metropolitan areas with high levels of alcohol-related problems have insufficient funds, while some of the shire counties are under spent (see above and MacGregor *et al.* 1993b). These disparities in funding distort the market.

There are also problems of access for various disadvantaged groups, like homeless offenders and the most vulnerable, chaotic clients. MacGregor *et al.* (1993a: 14) found that 24 per cent of those referred to residential services were homeless. There was concern that many homeless clients might be excluded in future, as a result of disputes over their residence qualifications between local authorities. Some authorities also reported that they would not reconsider chaotic clients who relapsed several times and needed repeated admissions to residential facilities. Both the geographical distribution of services and the disparities in funding create problems of access, therefore, as do user characteristics like homelessness and relapse. If permitted to continue, this would breach one of the cardinal principles of the original NHS: equality of access for those in equal need.

To summarise: the community care reorganisation could lead to a number of benefits for alcohol services. The overall philosophy of community care is normalisation, and this could help end the stigmatisation and marginalisation of people with alcohol problems, and of those who work with them. Pressure from the purchasing authorities for more cost-effective services could be positive, provided it does not end up restricting innovation and choice. There is a risk, however, that the contracting process could hinder the creativity of the independent sector, and that imperfections in the new market for social care could limit access to services by geographical location, social disadvantage or severity of problems. There is also a major problem over the administration costs that the new arrangements impose on local authorities. Conducting assessments for residential care is an expensive bureaucratic exercise, and in at least one case has led to an unanticipated reduction in community services.

The independent residential sector is also experiencing difficulties in this transitional period, largely because the funding mechanisms were not designed with alcohol services in mind. Provision of residential treatment and rehabilitation is at odds with the principles underpinning the government's community care policy. This is because, conceptually, *residential* is the opposite of *community*; and, second, because even if this were not the case the existing residential services are not usually local. This is symptomatic, in turn, of a larger problem, which is the way in which, increasingly, policy on alcohol treatment is constrained by a hostile policy environment; that is by the government's overriding concern to introduce market-based reforms in the health and social services. In the following section we consider the changing nature of the alcohol policy process, and the implications this has for future service development.

THREE AGES OF ALCOHOL POLICY

It is possible to identify three phases in the development of UK alcohol policy. In the first, dated from approximately 1951–74, policy-making was a bottom-up process. The initiative came from senior psychiatric consultants who were able to influence policy formation within the Ministry of Health. While many are critical of the incremental nature of health policy at this time, it is important to remember that the development of the alcohol field would have been considerably retarded were it not for the agenda-setting activities of concerned professionals. As Robinson and Ettorre (1980) show, there was a relatively rapid response within the NHS to the memoranda on the treatment of alcoholism, resulting in the establishment of a network of inpatient units, some of which had well-developed research and training functions.

In the second phase, dating from 1975, the policy process was interactive. Alcohol policy was guided by an informed professional consensus, with the health departments employing the mechanism of advisory committees to conduct systematic policy reviews. Research shaped the policy agenda, with a shift in emphasis from alcohol dependence to a broad range of alcohol problems; from treatment to prevention; and from hospital to community-based services. The growth of community provision was particularly marked in England, with the number of health districts lacking a rudimentary alcohol service falling from sixty in 1989 to four in 1994 (Alcohol Concern 1994). This was largely due to the activities of Alcohol Concern, established in 1983 as a national agency with the remit, amongst other things, to support local services and train voluntary counsellors.

There has been a gradual shift towards a less consultative policy process since the election of the Conservative government in 1979, but 1990 serves as a landmark with the passing of the National Health Service and Community Care Act. In this third phase, alcohol policy is characterised by a top-down process. Policy is now under firm political direction, with clinicians expected to advise on the best way to implement government strategies. This is in line with the managerial revolution in the NHS that accompanied the introduction of internal markets. Government still employs health professionals in an advisory capacity, but it is likely to be in a task force with carefully defined terms of reference, such as the one set up in 1994 to review services for drug misusers (Department of Health 1994). Rather than research determining the direction of policy, the purpose of research is to supply information in support of government strategy (see, e.g., Lord President's Office 1994: para 1.13).

These changes to the nature of the policy process may make it harder to rectify the problems with the government's community care policy. It is fashionable to be critical of the self-interest of the health professions, but the decline of professional influence over the direction of alcohol policy could have extremely negative consequences. Responsibility for alcohol policy spans many departmental boundaries. It is liable to fragmentation and is particularly constrained by the policy environment, that is by the broader sectoral policies adopted by government in relation to public expenditure, health, social services and criminal justice (Harrison and Tether 1987). There is a need for an efficient feedback and coordinating mechanism to prevent sectoral policies being adopted without regard for their impact on alcohol problems.

In the mid-1980s, government responded to criticism of policy coordination (see, for example, Harrison 1986) by establishing an Inter-Ministerial Group on Alcohol Misuse. This group no longer exists, and the regional alcohol coordinators established by the Department of Health may not survive the abolition of regional health authorities in 1995. It is hard to escape the conclusion that in the third age of alcohol policy, government has withdrawn from consultation and service planning and intends to let coordination be achieved by the 'invisible hand' of the market. Past experience suggests this will not be a successful strategy in the alcohol field.

REFERENCES

Alaszewski, A. and Harrison, L. (1992) 'Alcohol and social work: a literature review', *British Journal of Social Work*, 22(3): 331–343.

Alcohol Concern (1987) *Alcohol Services – The Future*, London: Alcohol Concern.

Alcohol Concern (1994) *Access to Alcohol Services*, London: Alcohol Concern.

Clement, S. (1987) 'The Salford experiment: an account of the Community Alcohol Team approach', in T. Stockwell and S. Clement (eds) *Helping the Problem Drinker: New Initiatives in Community Care*, London: Croom Helm.

Davies, D. L. (1979) 'Services for alcoholics', in M. Grant and P. Gwinner (eds) *Alcoholism in Perspective*, London: Croom Helm.

Department of Health (1989) *Caring For People: Community Care in the Next Decade and Beyond*, Cm. 849, London: HMSO.

Department of Health (1993) *Alcohol and Drug Services and Community Care*, LAC(93)2, London: Department of Health.

Department of Health (1994) *Task Force to Review Services for Drug Misusers*, 16 August, London: Department of Health.

Department of Health and Social Security (1973) *Community Services For Alcoholics*, Circular 21/73. London: DHSS.

Department of Health and Social Security (DHSS) (1975) *Better Services for the Mentally Ill*, Cm. 6233, London: HMSO.

Department of Health and Social Security and the Welsh Office (1977) *Prevention: Report of the Advisory Committee on Alcoholism*, London: DHSS.

Department of Health and Social Security and the Welsh Office (1978) *The Pattern and Range of Services for Problem Drinkers: Report of the Advisory Committee on Alcoholism*, London: HMSO.

Department of Health and Social Security and the Welsh Office (1979) *Education and Training for Professional Staff and Voluntary Workers in the Field: Report of the Advisory Committee on Alcoholism*, London: DHSS.

Druglink (1993) 'Report to DoH says community partnerships should replace district Drug Advisory Committees', *Druglink*, 8(6): 6.

Edwards, G. (1993) 'Substance misuse and the uses of science', in G. Edwards, J. Jaffe and J. Strang (eds) *Drugs, Alcohol and Tobacco: Making the Science and Policy Connections*, Oxford: Oxford University Press.

Glatt, M. (1974) *A Guide To Addiction and its Treatment*, Lancaster: Medical and Technical Publishing.

Glatt, M. (1982) *Alcoholism*, Sevenoaks: Hodder & Stoughton.

Harrison, L. (1986) 'Is a coordinated alcohol policy really feasible?', *Alcohol and Alcoholism*, 21(1): 5–7.

Harrison, L. and Tether, P. (1987) 'The coordination of UK policy on alcohol and tobacco: the significance of organisational networks', *Policy and Politics*, 15(2): 77–90.

Heather, N., and Robertson, I. (1989) *Problem Drinking*, Oxford: Oxford

University Press.

Holder, H., Longabaugh, R., Miller, W. R. and Rubonis, A. V. (1991) 'The cost effectiveness of treatment of alcoholism: a first approximation', *Journal of Studies on Alcohol*, 52(6): 517–40.

Home Office (1971) *Habitual Drunken Offenders: Report of the Working Party*, London: HMSO.

House of Commons (1992) *Parliamentary Debates (Hansard)*, Session 1992–93, 11 December, 215: 1177–84, London: HMSO.

House of Commons (1993) *Parliamentary Debates (Hansard)*, Session 1992–93, 8th June, 226: 128, London: HMSO.

Lord President's Office (1994) *Tackling Drugs Together*, CM. 2678, London: HMSO.

MacGregor, S., O'Gorman, A., Cattell, V., Flory, P., Savage, R. and Nelson, T. (1993a) *Who Cares Now?* London: Goldsmith College.

MacGregor, S., O'Gorman, A., Cattell, V., Flory, P. and Savage, R. (1993b) *Vulnerable Services for Vulnerable People*, London: Alcohol Concern and SCODA.

Ministry of Health (1962a) *A Hospital Plan For England and Wales*, Cm. 1604, London: HMSO.

Ministry of Health (1962b) *Hospital Treatment of Alcoholism*, Memorandum HM(62)43, London: Ministry of Health.

Ministry of Health (1968) *Treatment of Alcoholism*, Memorandum HM(68)37, London: Ministry of Health.

Ogden, J. (1992) 'Private home costs to soar predicts Labour', *Social Work Today* 23 (17): 4.

Orford, J. and Edwards, G. (1977) *Alcoholism: A Comparison of Treatment and Advice with a Study of the Influence of Marriage*, Oxford: Oxford University Press.

Robinson, D. and Ettorre, B. (1980) 'Special units for common problems: Alcoholism Treatment Units in England and Wales', in G. Edwards and M. Grant (eds) *Alcoholism Treatment in Transition*, London: Croom Helm.

Saunders, B. (1985) 'Counselling problem drinkers – research and practice', in J. Lishman (ed.) *Research Highlights in Social Work, Approaches to Addiction*, London: Kogan Page.

Shaw, S., Cartwright, A., Spratley, T. and Harwin, J. (1978) *Responding to Drinking Problems*, London: Croom Helm.

Spratley, T. A., Cartwright, A. K. J. and Shaw, S. J. (1975) *Designing a Comprehensive Community Response to Problems of Alcohol Abuse*, Report by the Maudsley Alcohol Pilot Project to the DHSS, London: Maudsley Hospital.

Spratley, T. A., Cartwright, A. K. J. and Shaw, S. J. (1977) 'Alcoholism: the changing role of the psychiatrist', in G. Edwards and M. Grant (eds) *Alcoholism: New Knowledge and New Responses*, London: Croom Helm.

WHO (1951) World Health Organisation Expert Committee on Mental Health: *Technical Report No. 42*, World Health Organization: Geneva.

Index